MEDICAL SCHOOL
from
HIGH SCHOOL

MEDICAL SCHOOL
from
HIGH SCHOOL

The College Applicant's Guide
to Medical School Early
Admission Programs

A.M. ILYAS, MD

Writers Club Press
San Jose New York Lincoln Shanghai

Medical School from High School
The College Applicant's Guide to Medical School Early Admission Programs

Writers Club Press
an imprint of iUniverse, Inc.

For information address:
iUniverse, Inc.
5220 S. 16th St., Suite 200
Lincoln, NE 68512
www.iuniverse.com

ISBN: 0-595-22725-2

Printed in the United States of America

I would like to take this opportunity to say thank you to two people that do not get to hear this often enough, my parents Qazi & Sajda Ilyas. They have provided my sisters and I with boundless love, support, and guidance. Without them I would not be whom I am today nor in the position to write this book.

To my wife, Erum, I cannot praise God enough for bringing you into my life. You have given my life such meaning and direction. With you next to me, I truly feel as though there is nothing I cannot achieve. It is only because of you that this book was ever completed.

CONTENTS

PROGRAM PROFILES

<u>*Undergraduate Institution*</u>

<u>*Medical Institution*</u>

Alabama

University of South Alabama

University of South Alabama College of Medicine

California

University of California—Riverside

University of California—
    Los Angeles School of Medicine

University of California—San Diego

University of California—
    San Diego School of Medicine

University of Southern California

University of Southern California—
    Keck School of Medicine

Connecticut

University of Connecticut

University of Connecticut School of Medicine

District of Columbia

George Washington University (7-year)

George Washington University School of Medicine

George Washington University (8-year)

George Washington University School of Medicine

Howard University

Howard University College of Medicine

Florida

University of Florida

University of Florida College of Medicine

University of Miami (6-year)

University of Miami School of Medicine

University of Miami (7-year)

University of Miami School of Medicine

Illinois

Illinois Institute of Technology

Finch University of the Health Sciences—
    Chicago Medical School

Illinois Institute of Technology

Rush Medical College

Northwestern University

Northwestern University Medical School

University of Illinois at Chicago

University of Illinois at Chicago College of Medicine

Indiana

Indiana State University

Indiana University School of Medicine

Undergraduate Institution	*Medical Institution*
Massachusetts	
Boston University	Boston University School of Medicine
Boston University	University of Medicine and Dentistry of New Jersey— New Jersey Medical School
Michigan	
Michigan State University	Michigan State University College of Human Medicine
University of Michigan	University of Michigan Medical School
Missouri	
University of Missouri—Kansas City	University of Missouri— Kansas City School of Medicine
New Jersey	
The College of New Jersey	University of Medicine and Dentistry of New Jersey— New Jersey Medical School
Drew University	University of Medicine and Dentistry of New Jersey— New Jersey Medical School
Montclair State University	University of Medicine and Dentistry of New Jersey— New Jersey Medical School
New Jersey Institute of Technology	University of Medicine and Dentistry of New Jersey— New Jersey Medical School
Richard Stockton College of New Jersey	University of Medicine and Dentistry of New Jersey— New Jersey Medical School
Rutgers University—Newark	University of Medicine and Dentistry of New Jersey— New Jersey Medical School
Rutgers University	University of Medicine and Dentistry of New Jersey— Robert Wood Johnson Medical School
Stevens Institute of Technology	University of Medicine and Dentistry of New Jersey— New Jersey Medical School
New York	
Binghamton University	State University of New York— Upstate Medical University College of Medicine
Brooklyn College	State University of New York— Downstate Medical Center College of Medicine
New York University	New York University School of Medicine
Rensselaer Polytechnic Institute	Albany Medical College
University of Rochester	University of Rochester of Medicine and Dentistry
Siena College	Albany Medical College
Sophie Davis School of Biomedical Education	City University of New York Medical School

Undergraduate Institution	_Medical Institution_
State University of New York—Stony Brook	State University of New York—Stony Brook School of Medicine Health Science Center
Union College	Albany Medical College

Ohio

University of Akron	Northeastern Ohio Universities College of Medicine
Case Western Reserve University	Case Western Reserve University School of Medicine
University of Cincinnati	University of Cincinnati College of Medicine
University of Dayton	University of Cincinnati College of Medicine
John Carroll University	University of Cincinnati College of Medicine
Kent State University	Northeastern Ohio Universities College of Medicine
Miami University	University of Cincinnati College of Medicine
Ohio State University	Ohio State University College of Medicine and Public Health
Xavier University	University of Cincinnati College of Medicine
Youngstown State University	Northeastern Ohio Universities College of Medicine

Pennsylvania

Drexel University	MCP Hahnemann School of Medicine
Lehigh University	MCP Hahnemann School of Medicine
MCP Hahnemann University	MCP Hahnemann School of Medicine
Monmouth University	MCP Hahnemann School of Medicine
Muhlenberg College	MCP Hahnemann School of Medicine
Pennsylvania State University	Jefferson Medical College
Rosemont College	MCP Hahnemann School of Medicine
Temple University	Temple University School of Medicine
Ursinus College	MCP Hahnemann School of Medicine
Villanova University	MCP Hahnemann School of Medicine
West Chester University	MCP Hahnemann School of Medicine
Widener University	Temple University School of Medicine
Wilkes University	MCP Hahnemann School of Medicine
Wilkes University	Pennsylvania State University College of Medicine
Wilkes University	SUNY – Upstate Medical University College of Medicine

Rhode Island

Brown University	Brown University School of Medicine
Providence College	Brown University School of Medicine
Rhode Island College	Brown University School of Medicine
University of Rhode Island	Brown University School of Medicine

Undergraduate Institution	_Medical Institution_
Tennessee	
East Tennessee State University	East Tennessee State University
	James H. Quillen College of Medicine
Fisk University	Meharry Medical College
Texas	
Rice University	Baylor College of Medicine
Texas A&M University	Texas A&M University College of Medicine
Virginia	
The College of William & Mary	Eastern Virginia Medical School
Hampden-Sydney College	Eastern Virginia Medical School
Old Dominion University	Eastern Virginia Medical School
Virginia Commonwealth University	Virginia Commonwealth University
	School of Medicine
Wisconsin	
University of Wisconsin	University of Wisconsin Medical School

FOREWORD

Here's a riddle…let's say two high school students enter a contest to see who the better golfer is at the end of one month. Both of these students are smart, work hard, have similar athletic abilities, and have never touched a golf club before. Now, let's say one of these students is not allowed to receive any golfing instruction (no coaches, no books, no videotapes, just "trial and error"). The other student is permitted daily teaching sessions from a golf pro, and is given numerous instruction books and videotapes. At the end of one month, who will win the contest? Obviously, the student with the professional instruction will be better prepared. The central theme to this riddle much like Dr. Ilyas's book *Medical School from High School,* is that being smart and working hard may get you to a certain point, but imagine how much farther you can strive with the right guidance and preparation.

No, the title of Dr. Ilyas's book is not a misprint. You can attend college without being one of the 500,000 applicants competing for 16,000 medical school seats. Your future as a physician will not depend upon getting an A+ or 4.0 in every college class. You won't have to constantly wonder whether that envelope in your dormitory mailbox is a rejection letter from the medical school you just applied to. All of these things are within your reach because like Dr. Ilyas's title says, you can indeed be admitted into medical school from high school. But, it's not going to happen to you by chance. It won't be because you obtained the highest SAT score in your school, or because you are on your way to becoming valedictorian. It won't be because you were voted president of the senior class, or captain of the wrestling team. The most crucial element in being admitted into any Medical School Early Admission Programs is…*being informed.*

Just like learning to golf, getting into medical school takes some coaching, and getting into medical school from high school requires even more coaching. Up till now, being informed wasn't so simple, there was no objective source of advice a high school student interested in becoming a physician could turn to, and no comprehensive list of Medical School Early Admission Programs available. Dr. Ilyas's work changes that, and makes being informed as easy as flipping the pages in his book.

A former US president used to say, "I don't mind surprises, the harder I prepare, the less surprised I get." Don't be surprised when it comes to your future as a physician. Don't make the mistake too many students do by whimsically saying "I'll go to college, apply, and hopefully I'll get into med school." Chance always favors a prepared mind. Let Dr. Ilyas's book *Medical School Admission from High School: The College Applicant's Guide to Medical School Early Admission Programs* be the first step in preparing you for a successful career as a physician.

Sean N. Higginson, MD
Mallinckrodt Institute of Radiology
Washington University
St. Louis, MO

PREFACE

To practice medicine is perhaps one of the greatest privileges society can offer an individual. For this reason, it is not surprising that competition for medical school admission is perennially so great. Based on this, it is astonishing how the topic of Medical School Early Admission Programs is foreign to most. Unfortunately, these programs have found themselves relatively unknown due to their obscure nature and from a lack of a universal title. In reality, Medical School Early Admission Programs are a wonderfully enriching and expeditious avenue for a committed high school student to pursue a career in medicine. It is my hope that with this book, more individuals undaunted by hard work and committed to joining the admirable field of medicine may increase their chances of becoming physicians.

My own perspective comes not only from my personal experiences of applying and being accepted to multiple Medical School Early Admission Programs, but also from the experience I gained by advising my siblings, relatives, and friends into obtaining admission into these programs. Throughout the years, I have amassed a considerable database of information on these programs. In addition, while in medical school I had the opportunity to act as a student admissions interviewer as well as a student ambassador. These experiences allowed me to understand the point of view of admission's personnel in addition to a student's.

Allow me to end this preface by saying that I have made every effort to be as diligent as possible in conveying the most accurate information to you, the reader. If there are any discrepancies, I strongly encourage you to contact me so changes can be made in future editions. In addition, I ask students, deans, and program advisers to contact me if there are any changes to the currently included programs, listed in Part B, or if any new programs have been started so I can add them to future editions. I can be reached at *EarlyMed@yahoo.com*.

In short, I believe this book is a must have for any high school student committed to a career in medicine and a mandatory reference book for every high school and college career guidance office in the country. If this resource helps even one college applicant committed to becoming a physician to gain admission to one of the many wonderful Medical School Early Admission Programs, my time has been well spent.

A. M. ILYAS, MD

Part A

CHAPTER 1

INTRODUCTION

"Medical School Early Admission Program?"

Medical School Early Admission Programs are guaranteed acceptance programs where students are simultaneously admitted to an undergraduate college as well as to a medical school directly from high school. Thereby, students begin college with the early assurance of acceptance to medical school. These programs arose in the 1960's and were designed to provide talented and motivated high school students interested in medicine an accelerated route to becoming a physician. The motivation was to offset the period's decline in the number of available physicians, due to the war effort, as well as due to the decline in the number and quality of applications to medical school. Decades later, these programs have persisted and prospered.

Since its inception, the number of Medical School Early Admission Programs have grown dramatically. Today, they exist under a vast array of titles. Yet, during this period of a few decades the number and quality of applications to medical schools has also grown dramatically. Then, why have these programs persisted, and increased for that matter, you might ask? The answer is that the experiment of accepting high school students preemptively to medical school resulted in other unforeseen benefits. It allowed local undergraduate and medical schools to recruit

and keep intelligent, motivated, and dedicated students before potentially losing them to other competing institutions. It also provided an
avenue to cultivate young minds by protecting them from the distraction and rigor of traditional medical school admissions. These minds
could now be free to contribute freely to their community, pursue
research, or simply pursue other areas of study not otherwise possible
for the traditional premedical student. In addition, some programs
evolved to address particular needs of various geographic locales, especially the shortage of primary care physicians in rural areas.

"What's the benefit?"

Traditionally, to go to medical school a student has to graduate from
high school, go onto college, take the MCAT, and then apply to medical
school during their junior year of college. This avenue represents the
vast majority of applications to medical school, generally 400,000 to
500,000 applications annually, as per the American Association of
Medical Colleges. Annually. These almost 500,000 applicants are vying
for about 16,000 seats in the country's 125 medical schools... stagger-
ing competition to say the least.

The benefits are obvious. A student seeking early admission, once having
met the requirements of the specific program, is competing within a considerably smaller applicant pool. Another major benefit of early admission is the decreased level of stress and anxiety. You have graduated high
school and have just begun college with a one-way ticket to medical
school before you have even walked into "Biology 101: The Cell."

"How does it work?"

The nuances of the application process will be detailed in Chapter 3, "Understanding the Application Process". Each Medical School Early Admission Program has individual requirements that are also outlined in detail in Part B of the book, "Program Profiles". In short, applicants apply to the individual undergraduate institution sponsoring a program as seniors in high school (Note: a few programs allow their students to apply after they are college freshman or sophomores). If they meet the program's requirements (ie, SAT scores, GPA, Rank, extra-curricular activities, all of which will be discussed in detail in later chapters) they will be invited for a formal interview. Once accepted into a program, the student will either spend 2, 3, or 4 years at the undergraduate institution (depending on the specifics of that program) before moving on to the respective medical school. While in college, the students will have to maintain a minimum GPA, may or may not be required to achieve a minimum score on the MCAT, and participate in various enrichment programs. Again, all of the specifics of the programs are outlined in Part B of the book.

"Knowledge & Effort is everything."

Before we go any further, allow me to define the most important underlying principle of how to successfully achieve acceptance to Medical School Early Admission Programs or any professional aspiration in general, for that matter: Success does not lie in being the smartest—it lies in being the hardest working and the most informed.

I can share many stories of my peers that were exceptionally intelligent but lacked either the motivation to work hard or the correct information to guide them. Fortunately, I have more stories of determined individuals undaunted by hard work and committed to knowing "the how," who have gone on to do great things.

If you are a student reading this book, you are clearly on the road to becoming informed. Now, if you are committed to a career in medicine and are willing to work as hard as necessary, then join me as we discuss the specifics of getting into medical school from high school.

CHAPTER 2

MEDICAL SCHOOL EARLY ADMISSION Q&A's

In order to help explain the nature of Early Admission Medical Programs in further detail, I have decide to use this chapter as a question and answer forum to respond to some of the most common questions I have encountered over the years.

- "How do Medical School Early Admission Programs work?"

As a preface, all of the details of the application process will be discussed in Chapter 3: "Understanding the Application Process," as well as further discussions on the various components of the application in chapters thereafter. In short, applying to Early Admission Programs is initially no different than applying to colleges traditionally. As a high school senior, you will submit the traditional college applications and note that you are applying for the institution's Medical School Early Admission Program. Additional application requirements may then be needed. For example, there may be specific supplemental applications or essays to complete. Also, additional paperwork may be requested such as additional letters of recommendation, SAT II scores, or details of activities you may have taken part in. After having applied and prior to acceptance into a program, you will be requested to appear for an interview at the participating medical school and/or the sponsoring

undergraduate institution to discuss your ambition of becoming a doctor, as well as to assess your character and maturity.

Once accepted into an Early Admission Program, you will begin your
education in the sponsoring undergraduate institution. The number of
years and credits you will be required to complete vary from program to
program. Generally the undergraduate component will consist of any-
where from two, three, or four years. During these undergraduate years,
you will fulfill the general requirements of your major. However, you
may have additional requirements such as maintaining a minimum GPA
and/or achieving a particular minimum MCAT score. In addition, Early
Admission students enjoy special benefits. Aside from the priceless peace
of mind that comes from knowing that you hold a seat in medical
school, these students participate in various enrichment experiences
geared at preparing them for a career in medicine.

Following the completion of the assigned number of undergraduate
years and/or credits, and meeting the minimum GPA and/or MCAT
requirements, you will be promoted to the respective medical school.
Once matriculated into medical school, your requirements as an Early
Admission student will be no different from those of any other medical
student. The length of the medical school portion of your education
will be the standard four years, after which you will be awarded the
Doctor of Medicine degree.

- "What's in it for me?"

Applying from high school allows you to avoid competing with the
almost 500,000 annual college pre-medical student applications to
medical school. Therefore, although applying for fewer available

Medical School Early Admission Program seats, you will now be competing within a much smaller and very select applicant pool.

Once accepted into such a program, the greatest benefit is the peace of mind. For those who are unaware, the pre-medical student's undergraduate career is extremely competitive, rigorous, and at times, overwhelming. As an accepted student, you have the benefit of avoiding the stress and heartache of traditional admissions and the time to pursue your own academic and extra-curricular interests. In addition, Medical School Early Admission Programs generally sponsor various experiences to help prepare you for a career in medicine. Such experiences include shadowing physicians of various specialties to participating in cutting-edge medical research.

In addition, there are other benefits enjoyed by students accepted by Early Admission Medical Programs. These students are generally admitted into the college's "Honors Program", which provides an array of added benefits. For example, you may enjoy the luxury of taking special or limited enrollment courses, and you may be granted special improved housing accommodations.

Finally, one of the greatest benefits of being accepted into a Medical School Early Admission Program is a financial one. Early Admission students, like their "Honors Program" peers generally enjoy significant financial rewards in the form of merit-based scholarship and grants, particularly at private undergraduate institutions. Colleges provide this money as a means to entice well-qualified applicants to join their institution. The amounts obviously vary, but as an accepted student, you can be confident to receive some merit-based scholarship money.

- "Should I pass on an Ivy League college?"

This is a very individual question. However, what I can offer is a perspective on the competitiveness of traditional medical school admissions and what an Ivy League or any prestigious undergraduate institution can offer. Getting accepted into medical school is extremely difficult whether you are applying from a prestigious or from a less-known institution. However, there are certain pros and cons when applying from prestigious institutions.

Prestige inherently offers the weight of an institution's name and history as a benefit. Also, the strong "network" or "connections" of a prestigious institution may prove to be an advantage to the pre-medical applicant. These connections result from the institution's varied alumni and age-old professional relationships. Also, prestigious institutions tend to have greater resources for its students in terms of coursework, research, and extra-curricular opportunities.

On the other hand, disadvantages also exist for pre-medical students applying from these prestigious institutions. Pre-medical students at these colleges are often lulled into a false sense of security that the institutions "name" will "get them in," and lesser credentials, grades, or MCAT scores will suffice. Also, competition tends to be quite fierce. These students are competing against highly intelligent and motivated peers for a limited number of "A's" in their courses. In addition, you may also be competing with a greater number of fellow pre-medical students for the attention of the faculty members, letters of recommendation, or research opportunities.

I should note that the pros and cons I have mentioned apply to the pre-medical students. These rules do not carry across all the different majors. One last point to consider when deciding between a Medical

School Early Admission Program or a more prestigious undergraduate institution where you would embark on the traditional pre-medical route, is to realize that your undergraduate education is just one step. It is not the ultimate goal of your education. By the time you become a physician you will have graduated from high school, then college, then medical school, and eventually, from a residency. Therefore, if it is a doctor you wish to be, focus on which college or program is best suited to facilitate this end goal.

- **"Can I change my mind about being a doctor after I've started?"**

Absolutely. There are no contracts signed when you begin an Early Admission program. Although not desired by admissions personnel, it is expected that some accepted students will change their career aspirations during their undergraduate career. That is the inherent beauty of college. It is a period of personal and professional discovery. But, the application process is designed to select students strongly committed to a career in medicine. Hence, the number of students leaving such programs willfully tends to be low.

- **"Am I sacrificing the length of my undergraduate experience?"**

First off, Medical School Early Admission Programs come in various lengths. Certain programs are accelerated, where you will spend only two or three years in college, while other programs incorporate a full un-accelerated four years of college. In addition, programs vary in the number of credits that a student has to complete before being promoted to medical school. In short, programs come in various shapes and forms. Each are tailored to fit a particular mold to meet the program's goals as well as to attract specific students. As an applicant, you are in position to choose the program that fits your needs and wishes the best.

Most students who have participated in Early Admission programs will tell you that "sacrificing" is actually the exact opposite of their experience. Rather, as mentioned earlier, these students are privy to an array of benefits and advantages while in college that only enrich their overall experience.

- **"Will I still have a well-rounded undergraduate experience?"**

Definitely. I would venture to say more so. The reason is quite simple, you have time and the peace of mind to venture out, try different things, and participate in activities and organizations that you may not otherwise have had the time to do. You do not have the distraction of the rigors associated with being a traditional pre-medical student. Also, you will see as you read Part B, "Program Profiles," that most program's provide and encourage their student's to participate in various enrichment experiences meant to challenge as well as prepare them for a career in medicine.

- **"Is it right for me?"**

Again, this is an individual question. I have tried in this chapter to highlight commonly asked features of Medical School Early Admission Programs through a question & answer forum. However, this discussion assumes the underlying premise that you are committed to a career in medicine. If you are unsure about becoming a physician, then these programs may not be right for you. Therefore, it is first most important to identify your career goal if possible. From there, you must determine what route you would like to take. As in all situations, it is helpful to speak to people older than you for advice who have experienced what you question. In the end, it is your decision alone.

For those still committed to attaining acceptance into Medical School Early Admission Programs, let's continue our discussion and delve into the details of the application process and the components of your credentials.

CHAPTER 3

UNDERSTANDING THE APPLICATION PROCESS

Applying to Medical School Early Admission Programs is initially the same as applying to college, with one exception. For those high school students committed to attaining medical school admission from high school, preparation must begin much earlier than filling out the application during senior year.

"Through the Admission Counselor's eyes"

In order to optimize your efforts, you must first understand what an Admission Counselor sees when he/she examines your application. Although you may consider certain aspects of your application to be your strengths, the Admission Counselor may judge your application with different priorities. Therefore, the best way for you to ensure a competitive application is by examining your credentials in the manner an Admission Counselor would when your application arrives on his/her desk.

The order of importance of high school credentials from the Admissions Counselor point of view is :

(1) SAT
(2) Rank/GPA
(3) Interview
(4) Extra-Curricular Activities (school, community, and medical)

Please do not be disheartened by this rank list. Read on and I will elaborate on the details of this order of importance. The underlying premise is understanding the importance of your various credentials can be the vital difference distinguishing an average and a
"shoe-in" applicant. With this information you can concentrate your energy where it counts the most and thereby buff your credentials in a manner to optimize your application.

"SAT ???...What about my Grades?"

It may shock or even upset you to hear that high SAT scores are more important than a good GPA, although your teachers and guidance counselors may have been telling you the contrary for many years. Allow me to explain how we are both correct, in relative terms.

The importance of the SAT, and the MCAT for that matter, stems from the fact that many medical school admission officers use these numbers as the primary cut-offs to decide which of the hundreds of applications will be evaluated. The simple reason is that they are the single most objective piece of data in your application. The SAT is a standardized exam. Therefore, every applicant takes the same exam, under the same conditions, and is graded on the same scale. The scores on these tests give the best indication of how an applicant matches up with his or her peers regardless of other parameters.

Your high school GPA and Rank are a close second to your SAT scores. The difference lies in their inherent subjectivity. High school grades are subjective due to variations in coursework difficulty, instruction, grading, and peer competition. Consequently, the SAT provides Admission Counselors a single objective score to quickly compare and distinguish between applicants. In addition, undergraduate and medical school Admission Counselors are very keen at analyzing a high school transcript and determining the level of difficulty of the individual student's curriculum as well as the high school's curriculum as a whole. Therefore, in defense of every teacher we have had that has pushed us to work hard at our grades, working hard not only helps us attain good grades, but also prepares us for standardized exams, such as the SAT. There will be more discussion on the SAT and Grades in Chapters 3 and 4, respectively. Another caveat to consider, undergraduate Admissions Counselors have more leeway in considering applicants for regular admissions. In this traditional circumstance applications are less susceptible to pre-weeding with SAT scores alone, and therefore, are more comprehensively evaluated.

"Interview!...What do I talk about?"

Again, we will discuss the "in's and out's" of the medical school interview in detail ahead in Chapter 6. For now, I would like to acknowledge that for a high school student, an interview for a Medical School Early Admission School Program will most likely be their first "professional" interview. Generally, applicants applying to colleges do not have to interview. All medical school admissions however require interviews. At this junction, I wish to only leave you with three words to think about until we arrive at Chapter 6: Confidence, Maturity, and Commitment. These are the attributes you must embody at your interview. We'll talk more about this in Chapter 6.

"Should I volunteer at a local hospital?"

Absolutely!!! This is extremely crucial. Again, I did not wish to discourage applicants by saying that SAT and grades are more important than extra-curricular activities. The importance of your SAT and grades is to make the initial cuts. Once you make the cut, then your application is opened up and examined and that is when your activities become vital. The activities that I am alluding to are those in addition to normal school activities. It is important to illustrate your interest and commitment to medicine by the activities in which you partake inside and outside of school. On paper, your activities provide you with the personal commitment to medicine that you need to convey. During the interview, your activities provide you with the material you will want to discuss.

"Let's discuss this in more detail…"

The activities you pursue in your community will be strongly scrutinized. Virtues that Admission Counselors will peruse for is a commitment to community service, involvement in health related activities, and participation in leadership roles. They seek these virtues because these are the virtues that society seeks in a physician.

Therefore, don't quit your mall job. Rather, consider also working as a camp counselor or volunteering in a local hospital, medical clinic, or nursing home. These activities are mutually beneficial. It allows you to contribute to your community in a tangible venue while also allowing you to learn more about real life medicine. Other suggestions include training as an EMT, volunteering in an ER, learning/teaching CPR, and volunteering for the Red Cross. Community service with a medical or community health tone is a key component to your application. Often, the demonstration of some involvement in the medical arena is a pre-requisite for many programs.

"What about the school play?"

Just like everything else, it is important to recognize the significance of extra-curricular activities in school. Being active in school activities and clubs is essential. Although, what you actually do and the amount of time you actually commit to these activities is not always the priority of Admission Counselors. Their concern is to determine how well-rounded and active you have been. Participating in extra-curricular activities is a great way to be a part of one's school community. It is a healthy and productive outlet for your energy, abilities, and talents. It is a way to express your intellectual, organizational, and social skills. It is a way of making friends, contacts with members of the community, and getting to know your school faculty. And, at the very least, it is fun.

Sports, just as school clubs, illustrate how well-rounded you are. School sports, however, can provide an added advantage if you are a recognized athlete in a particular sport. Another benefit is the opportunity to inter-view with an individual that shares the same enthusiasm for a sport as you. These are wonderful circumstances that can make your application stand out and provide opportunities to personally relate with your interviewer during the interview.

School clubs, particularly nationally recognized ones, are excellent organizations in which to be involved. Participating in student govern-ment provides an applicant with the opportunity to be a class leader and an avenue to become recognized by school faculty and administra-tion. Honor societies are also excellent organizations in which to be involved, particularly since membership requires meeting certain prerequisite criteria. These honors inherently distinguish you from the rest of your class. Honor society membership proves that an applicant is a competitive and active student at his/her school as well as at the national level.

To reiterate, extra-curricular activities, including school sports and clubs as well as community activities are vital to your application by making you a well-rounded applicant. I will leave you with one warning: participating in activities should never occur at the expense of your grades. Remember, no grades means no interview. Time management is key in maintaining good grades and also pursuing your extra-curricular interests.

"The main course"

Allow me to leave you with this metaphor: consider your application as a meal being served to an Admission Counselor at a restaurant. Your SAT and Rank/GPA are the main course. Your extra-curricular activities are the condiments, your interview the quality of service. Without the main course, the condiments and service are irrelevant. With bad service (poor interview), even great food is unpleasant.

CHAPTER 4

The SATs

SAT is the well-known acronym for the Scholastic Assessment Test. It is more specifically known as the SAT I—The Reasoning Test, and also affectionately known as the "College Boards," named so after the not-for-profit organization that has been administering the exam for over one hundred years. (There is also the SAT II—The Subject Tests, which will be discussed shortly).

The SAT I is a three-hour test made up of seven sections:

- Three **verbal** sections: two 30-minute sections and one 15-minute section.
- Three **math** sections: two 30-minute sections and one 15-minute section.
- One 30-minute **"equating"** section that is either verbal or math.

The verbal questions are designed to test your ability to: understand and analyze what you read, recognize relationships between parts of a sentence, and establish relationships between pairs of words. The math questions are designed to test your ability on: arithmetic, algebra, and geometry. The equating section is experimental and does not count towards your score. It is used by the College Boards to "test-out" questions to be used potentially on future exams.

The SAT is scored out of a maximum of 1600. The Verbal and Math sections count for a maximum score of 800 each. Test-takers start with a minimum score of 200 on each section. Therefore, potential scores can range from 400 to 1600 points.

For more logistical specifics on the SAT, refer to the College Board website: http://www.collegeboard.org/

"It's just one test!"

It is true that the SAT is only one exam. The reality, however, is that it can define a student academically. The reason is simple: it serves as the one true objective performance measure available to Admission Counselors. As discussed earlier, even though you spend every day working on your high school records, all of your grades are influenced by a certain degree of inherent subjectivity. Variations abound between differences in high school coursework difficulty, instruction, grading, and peer competition. The SAT controls for all that. The same exam is offered to every student, with the same level of difficulty, under the same conditions, and is graded the same. In addition to its objectivity, it also reflects how students prepare for and respond to a single significantly stressful situation.

"The SAT, the SAT, and the SAT"

If someone asked me what are the top three most important credentials in your application to a Medical School Early Admission Program, I would reply "first, the SAT, second, the SAT, and third, the SAT." It is unfortunate that a single exam carries so much weight, but as mentioned earlier, it is the single most objective qualifier of a student's ability. Don't be confused by this statement. The SAT's extreme importance stems from its above mentioned objective characteristics as well as its common use as the primary weeding tool in determining who is interviewed and who is not. However, admission to medical school cannot be secured without the other application components, such as grades and extra-curricular activities.

"Just the beginning of a long line of tests."

There is another nuance to the SAT as it relates to the field of medicine. Much weight is placed on the SAT for those students applying for early admission to medical school because the SAT is just the first in a long line of standardized exams that a student will have to take on the road to becoming a doctor. First there is the SAT in high school followed by the MCAT in college. In medical school there is the United States Medical Licensing Exam (USMLE) Step 1 and the USMLE Step 2. In residency there is the USMLE Step 3 as well as your specialty's Board Certification exam. Then, as a practicing physician, there are license-renewing exams every five or ten years, depending on the regulations of that time. Standardized-test taking ability is a well sought after trait in medical school applicants due to the testing demands of the medical field. Therefore, a student's performance on the SAT exam not only represents ability and preparedness, but it is also a yardstick to predict future performance on standardized exams.

"When should I take the SAT?"

High Schools generally recommend taking the SAT during the junior year and during the first semester of the senior year of high school, if necessary. Technically, there is no limit to when and how often you can take the exam. As a rule of thumb, although the exam can be taken more than once, taking it more than three times is frowned upon. Since most of you are intending on taking the SAT for the first time during the winter or spring of your junior year, preparation must begin well in advance. A good time to commence preparation is the summer between your sophomore and junior year, after you have received your PSAT scores.

The PSAT

In order to begin mapping out your SAT preparation, it is important to gauge one's baseline ability on the SAT for diagnostic purposes. One such opportunity is to take the PSAT during the sophomore year of high school. The PSAT is the acronym for the Practice Scholastic Assessment Test. It serves two purposes: to provide a run through and preview of the SAT, as well as to provide a platform for students to qualify for various scholarship and recognition programs, sponsored by the National Merit Scholarship Corporation. The PSAT is an abridged form of the SAT I and, therefore, is also designed to measure a student's critical reading, math problem-solving, and writing abilities. It is scored out of 160, with a maximum score of 80 on the Verbal and Math sections each. Hence the PSAT is based on one tenth of the scoring scale of the SAT I. The PSAT that is considered for scholarship purposes is the one offered in the fall of a student's junior year. Therefore, a great way to begin preparation for the SAT is by taking the PSAT during the sophomore year with the current juniors. It can serve as a diagnostic test and thereby provide information on your baseline ability under standardized conditions. It will also define how much work you have to do in order to reach your goal.

"But I thought you weren't supposed to study for the SAT?"

It astounds me to this day that some people still proclaim this notion. For the serious test-taker, the SAT *does* require preparation. If there is any doubt, all of the test-prep companies vying for your business will attest to the fact that preparation can definitely improve your score. Personally, I have yet to meet anyone whose exam scores did not improve with sincere preparation. At the very minimum, preparation provides a familiarity with the exam that alone can improve one's score by reducing anxiety if nothing else. Let's reiterate this point: test preparation will improve your score on the SAT, as well as for every standardized exam you will ever take.

SAT Preparation Suggestions:

Many resources are available for those seeking help with SAT preparation. Before mentioning some of the test preparation sources, allow me to share a few test-taking tips to help improve your score.

• **Questions, Questions, Questions!** : The quickest way to improve your score on the SAT, and on other standardized exams, is to do lots and lots of questions. Practicing a high volume of questions has multiple benefits: Reviewing the answers to questions in detail helps you understand the question-writer's logic and thought processes, which will permeate through future questions. It familiarizes you with commonly tested themes. It improves your timing and endurance. Lastly, it will decrease anxiety by increasing your familiarity and comfort level with the exam.

• **Time management** : Be conscious of the amount of time you spend on each question and the amount allotted to you for the section. Wear a watch during the exam. The best way to improve your endurance and time management, or your speed in answering questions is, again, by doing a lot of questions.

• **Avoid omitting** : The SAT is one of the few exams you will encounter that actually punishes you for getting the wrong answer. Specifically, you are penalized a quarter point. Therefore, guessing is formally discouraged. In reality, this penalization often results in a stigma where students are afraid to make educated guesses and cause them to believe that omitting is probably better than guessing. This is absolutely false. I am not suggesting that you guess at every question you have no clue about. I am recommending that if you can rule out at least one or two question choices, then make an educated guess. The benefit of guessing correctly in one out of every four guesses will improve your score more than just omitting four questions. If you speak with those students who score in the 13, 14, or 1500's you will learn that they avoid omitting questions because they need every point to attain their high scores. If you have absolutely no idea on a question, it is probably better to omit. If you can even rule out one or two options however, it is often worth taking an educated guess. Again, doing a large volume of practice tests will help define your skills in the process of elimination and the cost/benefit of omitting questions.

SAT Preparatory Resources

A slew of resources are available for SAT preparation. They vary considerably in price as well as in quality. Many classes and books are available, each with their own pros and cons. Below I have listed some well respected resources. Remember that many more qualified programs do exist. Also, remember that what works for some may not work for others. Determining which resource you would like to use, if any, depends on your own style of studying and learning needs. It is always a good idea to ask around, especially senior students, to see what worked for them. Books are always cheaper than courses. Courses typically run about $1000. That is a hefty sum of money. But, in the grand scheme of the amount of money you will commit to your undergraduate and medical education, the amount you spend on test preparation is just a drop in the bucket. At the very minimum, seek a good bank of practice questions. Question banks are available from test prep courses as well as from many books geared towards SAT preparation available in any local bookstore.

Below is a listing of some common test-prep courses and resources to start with:

- The College Boards: http://www.collegeboards.org/
- Kaplan: http://www.kaplan.com/
- Princeton Review: http://www.princetonreview.com/
- Scholastic Testing Service: http://www.testprep.com/
- College Power Prep: http://www.powerprep.com/
- Barron's: http://www.barronseduc.com/
- Peterson's: http://www.petersons.com/

The SAT II

The SAT II are subject tests. They are a collection of one hour exams covering a variety of subjects. They include: Literature, Writing, US History, World History, Mathematics, Biology, Chemistry, Physics, and a variety of Foreign Languages. The individual subject exams are one hour long and you can take up to three subject exams on one exam date. Each subject exam is scored out of a maximum score of 800. Again, preparation is necessary to excel on these exams as well. Good resources to use include the one's listed earlier. Preparation is even more critical for these since they test your factual knowledge on a specific topic, not just your reasoning abilities as in the SAT I. On the same token, it may be easier to prepare for these because they are topic-specific. As a rule of thumb, it is better to concern yourself with preparation for the SAT II after you have prepared for and successfully taken the SAT I. Dividing your time between preparation for both exams will prove counter-pro-ductive.

Many colleges require or recommend taking one or more of the SAT II subject tests for admission or placement. A variety of Medical School Early Admission Programs require SAT II subject tests. Please refer to Part B for specific SAT II requirements for the different programs.

CHAPTER 5

GPA / RANK

Your GPA and Rank are the summation of the first three years of high school, from freshman to junior year. Although senior grades also may come into play, generally college applications reflect grades through the junior year when initially submitted. Discussing the importance of attaining good grades goes without saying. Therefore, I won't bore you with what everyone has been telling you since kindergarten. Rather, let us discuss what Medical School Early Admission programs are looking for.

"A's and B's, right?"

Many of the Medical School Early Admission Programs have specific requirements for high school grades ranging from a minimum GPA of 3.0 to some that require a 4.0 in order to be considered. Since GPA requirements vary, just hold to the doctrine "higher the better." You should at minimum expect to maintain a 3.3-3.5, or at least a 90%. I believe that this is not unfair to ask of any serious student. As for rank, not every program considers a student's class rank. For those that do, rank requirements vary from requiring that a student rank in the top 25% to the top 5% of their high school class. Admission Counselors are well aware that not all schools rank their students. Therefore, they will consider your GPA alone in its place.

Although the fundamental principle to attaining good grades and a high rank is hard work, there are other steps that can be taken to improve one's credentials.

Honors, Gifted, & AP Courses

Many high schools offer courses that are weighted heavier than others due to a higher level of difficulty or special enrollment requirements. Common examples of these courses include Honors, Gifted, or Advanced Placement (AP) courses. In certain schools, these courses may be weighted with additional bonus points to be added to the earned grade when calculating the GPA. Whether or not a course is weighted must be determined at the individual high school registrar's office.

In addition to the advantage of their weighted status, such honors courses reflect positively on your transcript. Admission Counselors are keen at determining the difficulty of a student's high school course load. For example, they can appreciate the strength of a student who has earned a 3.4 taking predominantly Honors or AP courses versus a student who has a 3.7 GPA in all average to below average difficulty-level courses.

A word of warning, taking a weighted course may help bolster your GPA with additional points, but the courses are also generally more difficult. If you earn lower grades in these courses, taking them may overshadow the benefits. In addition, the grade that will appear on your transcript will be the un-weighted one. Therefore, when considering whether to take weighted courses, remember that it is always better to get an "A" in a regular course, than a "C" in a very difficult course. Be wise and carefully select your courses by assessing the intensity and considering your own ability and time. The best combination is taking all college-preparatory caliber courses with some weighted courses sprinkled in which you are confident that you can do well in.

Suggestions on Getting Good Grades

• **Review old questions/exams** : As mentioned earlier in the discussion of the SAT, the best preparation is always to do a lot of questions. That goes for your coursework as well. Some teachers will provide old tests for review. For those that do not, senior students are a good resource for old exams. Old exam questions are an invaluable asset. Unfortunately, if a teacher does not want you to see an old exam, he/she won't allow students to keep them. The premise of this type of review is simple. It allows you to familiarize yourself with the subject matter and the teacher's style of questioning. As you will quickly see, the themes that a teacher wishes to stress do not vary much from year to year.

• **Understand, don't memorize** : Understanding a concept is always more valuable than memorizing facts. Memorizing is generally considered to be the lowest form of intellect. There is a place for it, however. Every one must memorize certain things, especially doctors. But, whenever given the opportunity to learn something conceptually or theoretically, it is always worth your while to learn it rather than only memorizing the facts. We always retain concepts better than random facts.

• **Make your own notes/flashcards** : Most students study from a combination of a book and class notes. Making your own notes that highlight and review important points stressed in the book and class provide two major advantages. It provides a quick review source of material written in your own words and with your own understanding of the matter. Your own thoughts are generally better recollected than the thoughts of others. Second, it provides an exercise in physically writing down facts. Writing down or reiterating things is a form of reinforcement that helps you remember things.

- **Study alone:** Group studying, although fun, is often unproductive. Don't fall into the trap of studying in a group because of the theory that discussing and explaining a topic to another allows you to understand it better. It is true that teaching helps fortify your understanding as well as illustrate your grasp of a topic. But, the premise relies on the notion that you have actually learned the material prior to a discussion. Initially, it is best to learn a topic conceptually on your own, without the distractions of a social forum.

- **Have fun:** Remember the idiom, "All work and no play..." Working hard in high school, as well as in college and medical school requires a balance between work as well as leisure/personal/social time. You will always be more productive if you are happy, rested, and have some non-academic interests to pursue.

CHAPTER 6

THE INTERVIEW

Almost every Medical School Early Admission Program requires an interview. If you have been requested to appear for an interview, this means you have met all or most of a program's initial screening requirements (ie, SAT and Grades) and have now moved on to the next round. All applicants invited for an interview are generally on equal footing. Their performance at the interview coupled with their credentials will dictate who will ultimately receive an offer for admission. As a general rule of thumb, programs interview two to four times as many applicants as there are seats.

For most high school students, this will be your first professional interview. Interviews can be a scary and intimidating experience for many people. The best way to overcome anxiety regarding interviews is to know what to expect, how to prepare for it, and to understand what an interviewer wants.

Preparation & Practice

Allow me to preface this discussion on interviews by saying that not all good interviewees are "naturals." Rather, being able to interview well is an acquired trait that requires some preparation and practice. If you have reached the point of receiving invitations to interview for a seat in a Medical School Early Admission Program, you definitely have reason to improve your abilities. Just as the SAT is the first in a long line of standardized exams, so to is this interview the first in a long line of interviews you will give on the path to becoming a physician. Therefore, prepare for your interviews seriously. With time you will see that the more you interview, the more at ease you will become.

"Where am I going?"

First, understand what you are interviewing for. This may sound obvious enough, but you will be surprised how subtle it may truly be. Allow me to elaborate. Preparing for your interview means more than just knowing you are interviewing for medical school. Rather, it also means knowing all of the details of the specific program, knowing facts regarding the participating undergraduate and medical school, and being familiar with the professional background of your interviewers. For instance, it will be embarrassing to begin an interview and not know whether this program is an accelerated six-year program or a full eight-year program. On the same token, it is a faux pas to address your interviewer as "mister" or "misses" when they may more likely be "Dean," "Professor," and/or "Doctor."

"What will I say?"

Although it is impossible and impractical to have a prepared answer for every question, it is reasonable to be prepared to answer some very likely questions or scenarios. For example, here are some commonly asked questions:

- Tell me about yourself?
- Tell me about your family?

- When did you first decide you wanted to become a doctor?
- How did you come to the decision that medicine is for you?
- Was there one single experience that led you to the decision to become a doctor?
- What specialty of medicine would you like to practice?
- Do you see yourself as a primary care doctor or a specialist?
- What do you like to do in your free time?
- What is your favorite sport?
- What is the last book you read?
- Who is your favorite author?
- What do you believe is your greatest strength?
- What do you believe is your greatest weakness?
- What do you believe has been your greatest achievement to this point?
- What do you believe has been your greatest failure to this point?
- What is the most difficult decision you have ever had to make?
- What leadership positions have you held?
- What was your favorite class?
- Who was your favorite teacher and why?
- Who has had the greatest impact on you?
- Where do you see yourself professionally in 20 years?
- Tell me something about yourself that separates you from the other applicants?

The above are some very common medical school interview questions. There are certain questions you may receive that are specific to the

Medical School Early Admission Program that you are applying for. They may include questions like:

- What leadership roles have you assumed?
- How did you come to the decision you wanted to be a doctor?
- Why are you interested in Early Admission to medical school?
- What features attract you to our program?
- How will you benefit from an Early Admission program?
- Do your parent's want you to be a doctor?
- What hospital/medical-related experience have you had?
- How do you feel about working with sick and dying patients?
- If you do not gain Early Admission to medical school, what will you do?
- What can you contribute to our program/institution?

These are just a handful of questions that you may be asked. The point is not to have specific answers to every question, but rather be prepared to answer questions regarding the root of your interest in medicine, your future practice ambitions, details about personal experiences mentioned on your application, and what qualities and strengths you have to offer. At first, it is hard to talk about oneself because it feels unnatural to most of us under normal circumstances. An interview, however, is not a normal circumstance. It has its own rules, and the rule is to share your strengths and qualities eagerly and earnestly.

In addition to preparation for questions such as those posed above, be prepared to discuss current events. The interviewer will not be expecting a detailed summary of the latest international peace accords. However, they may be curious to see how well read and aware you are of such matters. In addition, health related topics are always popular. For example, common topics include:

- Do you believe doctors make too much money?

- Is free health care a right?

- How could we improve our nation's current health care disparities?

- Do you believe in national health insurance?

- Do you think health maintenance organizations are effective?

- How involved do you believe the government should be in health care?

- Do you believe abortion is a woman's right?

- What are your thoughts on Euthanasia?

- What do you believe is America's role in helping foreign countries in need?

- Do you think the president is doing a good job?

You may be thinking that these are tough and controversial questions . . . you are right! Understand that these are controversial questions because there is not always a right or wrong answer. If there were, there would be no controversy. The goal of an interviewer who asks controversial questions is to determine three things: (1) Are you familiar with the topic? (2) Are you able to formulate an argument and support it? And, (3) are you able to respond under pressure? They are not concerned with your particular belief, but rather how you can support and argue for that belief while maintaining your poise. One caveat, be mindful about expressing a personal belief that may be somewhat controversial in its own right. An interview for medical school is no time to be professing extreme opinions.

In addition to these controversial questions, be prepared for some questions intended to throw you off balance. Interviewers have been known to ask questions like, "Let's see who can do more push-ups." Or, "tell me a joke." Again, these questions are geared to see how you respond. Stay calm and respond professionally.

"What should I wear?"

When you walk in to the office for the interview, you want to exude the appearance of conservative clean-cut success. Men should wear a suit, dress shirt, and tie. A navy blue or black suit, with a subtle tie is a winning combination. Women should wear a conservative suit or dress. Again, navy blue or black is best. Keep the dress length at or below the knees. As much as an interviewer of the opposite sex may enjoy a provocative outfit, an interviewer of the same sex will not. This also goes for excessive make-up. Both sexes should appear polished and well groomed. Your clothing should be clean and free of wrinkles. Men should avoid growing a beard or mustache during their interview period, as well as trying out a new trendy haircut. If you already have a beard, make sure it is well trimmed. Avoid anything flashy. This is not the time to show off your fashionable wardrobe. Aim for clean-cut and professional.

"What else should I bring?"

Aside from your sharp clothes you should bring some paperwork along. Specifically, have a resume listing your name, contact information, high school information, SAT/Grades/Rank, honors achieved, leadership positions held, extra-curricular activities, and any employment information. In addition, bring a copy of your transcript with the latest grades and any recent achievements that may have occurred since the application was submitted. If you happened to have published something, bring a copy of the publication. In short, bring things that illustrate your academic and leadership prowess that pertain to you professionally.

"What do they want to see?"

The personality traits that an interviewer wants to see immediately and throughout the interview from you can be summed up in three words: confidence, maturity, and commitment.

• **Confidence** : This represents confidence without cockiness. You must display a sense of self-assurance when you talk about yourself and answer their questions. Your confidence will be tested as well as re-affirmed in the discussion of controversial topics. Again, they will not be concerned with your particular belief. Rather, they will want to observe your poise and ability to defend your position.

• **Maturity** : Can you hold an intellectual conversation with an older daunting professional without being intimidated? Can you handle yourself in a foreign environment with poise? Can you discuss a topic, handle criticism, and support a stance without being either too rigid or too agreeable? These are the subtle markers of maturity.

• **Commitment** : Specifically, do you convey an unrelenting passion and commitment to pursuing a career in medicine? The lack of commitment is probably the kiss of death for many strong applicants. Remember, although you may be confident and committed to a career in medicine, to them you are very young, inexperienced, and whimsical. They are making a big commitment to you, six to eight years to be specific, as well as a huge financial commitment. If you show any signs of doubt or hesitation about pursuing a career in medicine, you might as well have not come. They need to know beyond a shadow of a doubt that you wish to be a doctor above all else.

"What should I do at the end?"

At the end of the interview, you will be asked if you have any questions. The answer is an enthusiastic "Yes!" Asking questions when prompted displays your interest as well as preparedness. Have three to four intelligent questions ready. Again, be mindful of what you say. Do not ask any questions that may be construed as derogatory to the program or institution, or to any of their competitors. Also, do not ask any questions that may be inappropriate for the particular interviewer. For example, do not ask the chairperson of the department or program what is the easiest way to get back home. Save any logistical questions for the interview-day coordinator. Rather, ask appropriate and thoughtful questions that underlie your interest in the program. Examples include:

- What opportunities are there for students to participate in research?
- What opportunities are there for students to participate in community programs?
- Are there opportunities for Early Admission students to gain clinical exposure?

Once you are home, it is good form to send a short thank you letter to each individual with whom you have interviewed. The letter should be addressed appropriately to the interviewer, with proper notation of their status (ie, PhD or MD). It should be brief, thanking them for having taken the time to interview you. It should also include a quick sentence re-affirming your interest in their program. Later, if you experience any new events, honors, or achievements that may strengthen your application following your interview, send a letter to the program director describing them and again re-affirming your interest in the program.

Suggested Reading:

Carnegie, Dale. *How to Win Friends and Influence People*. Pocket Books: 1994. (ISBN: 0671723650)

Molloy, John. *Dress for Success*. Warner Books: 1988. (ISBN: 0446385522)

Utterback, Ann. *College Admissions Face to Face: Making the Most of Interviews and Campus Visits*. Seven Locks: 1989. (ISBN: 0932020720)

Part B

PREFACE TO THE PROGRAM PROFILES

The Program Profiles section represents the truly unique and invaluable portion of this book. Much of the mystique and lack of awareness of Medical School Early Admission Programs revolve around the fact that these programs are not well organized nor centralized. The annual *AAMC's Medical School Admission Requirements* provides the best published account of these programs. However, even their list is considerably incomplete.

In profiling the various Medical School Early Admission Programs I had to pursue extensive research. The profiling data presented in the following pages represents information compiled from online sources on the internet, the *AAMC's Medical School Admission Requirements: 2000-2001*, and from various program deans and advisors, in that order.

I would like to stress here, that this list is likely to be incomplete. Programs such as these detailed here are in a constant state of evolution. In addition, the parameters, goals, and requirements of these programs also change frequently with contract renegotiations between participating institutions. Therefore, I would like to reiterate that it is my sincere desire only to relate the most accurate data to the reader. In there so doing, I request of the reader, specifically the students and program advisors, to update me on any discrepancies, changes in program features, or on the creation of new programs. I will update any changes with diligence in future editions. I can be reached at: *EarlyMed@yahoo.com*

UNDERSTANDING THE PROGRAM PROFILES

Program categorization

Each program profile is broken up into sections to provide the most efficient presentation of data to the reader. The profiles are categorized by the undergraduate institution first, and the medical school second. You may see an undergraduate institution listed more than once. That is because some colleges have more than one program with the same or different medical schools. The same goes for medical schools. You will notice medical schools listed multiple times with different undergraduate institutions.

Contact Information

I have provided contact information for both institutions participating in the Early Admission program, when applicable. These addresses, phone numbers, and email addresses were retrieved from either the respective websites or the *AAMC's Medical School Admissions Requirements: 2000-2001.* As a generalization, it will be more efficient to contact the listed undergraduate office for additional program information. Whenever possible, I tried to include the information of those individuals holding positions directly responsible for overseeing the program. I intentionally excluded specific names of individuals heading various programs, and limited it to their titles. The logic being, individuals tend to turnover more frequently than positions do. Also in the contact information I tried to include program websites whenever possible. Throughout my research, I found the websites to be generally the most up to date. I know that most high school students are quite savvy with the internet. Therefore I would strongly encourage students to seek Medical School Early Admission Program information on the web.

Tuition

My tuition values represent the 1999-2000 school year, unless otherwise noted. The values are for tuition only, not including fees and room/board charges. I noted out-of-state tuition for non-residents whenever applicable, unless the program was limited to in-state residents only. The tuition values were attained from the *AAMC's Medical School Admissions Requirements: 2000-2001*, and *Peterson's 2001 Guide to Colleges*.

About the Medical School and the BA/BS-MD Program

Following the contact information, I included information on the medical school and then the program details. The program details, listed as "About the BA/BS-MD Program," provides as much succinct information possible regarding the goal, organization, and requirements of the program. Because every Medical School Early Admission Program has some particular motivation, I tried to provide the most defining characteristics of each program.

Program Features/Requirements Table

In the table on the bottom of each program profile page, I have provided the program's specific title, length, high school requirements, and application deadline. This quick reference section is designed to provide a quick-reference section for each program. Again, I have tried to be as specific and succinct in my "numbers" as possible.

Program Profiles

| Undergraduate Institution: | **University of South Alabama** |
| Medical School: | University of South Alabama College of Medicine |

Undergraduate Contact Information:	_Medical School Contact Information:_
Office of Admissions	Office of Admissions
University of Sourth Alabama	University of South Alabama – College of Medicine
Administrative Building – Room 182	Mobile, Alabama 36688
Mobile, Alabama 36688	(334) 460-7176
(334) 460-6141	(800) 872-5247
1999-2000 tuition: $2,841 ($5,481 for non-residents)	_1999-2000 tuition_: $7,000 ($14,000 for non-residents)

About the Medical School:

The College of Medicine at the University of South Alabama is a public institution founded in 1973. The average class size is 65 students.

About the BS-MD Program:

Students in the senior year of high school or recently graduated individuals who have not yet entered college are eligible. The program is open to both residents and non-residents of Alabama. Students accepted into the program must maintain a minimum GPA of 3.5, and a minimum GPA of 3.4 in the sciences and mathematics. The MCAT is required and students must score above the national average. An interview will be conducted with the students after the completion of 96 quarter hours to assess the student's academic performance and continued commitment to medicine.

Program Title	The Combined BS/MD Early Admissions Program.
Length of Program	8 years.
Number of Students	15
High School Requirements	GPA of 3.5 / 4.0, minimum required. ACT score of 28, minimum required.
Application Deadline	March 1.
MCAT Requirements	Yes. Must achieve a score above the national average.

Undergraduate Institution: **University of California—Riverside**
Medical School: University of California—Los Angeles
                               School of Medicine

Undergraduate Contact Information:	*Medical School Contact Information:*
Student Affairs Officer	Office of Admissions
Division of Biomedical Sciences	UCLA School of Medicine
University of California – Riverside	Box 957035
Riverside, CA 92521	Los Angeles, CA 90095
(908) 787-4333	(310) 825-6081
bmscil@ucracl.ucr.edu	
1999-2000 tuition: $3,747	*1999-2000 tuition*: $10,128
($13,551 for non-residents)	($19,932 for non-residents)
http://biomed.ucr.edu/	

About the Medical School:

The University of California—Los Angeles School of Medicine is a public institution situated on the main UCLA campus. It graduated its first medical school class in 1955. The average class size is 145 students.

About the BS-MD Program:

The Thomas Haider Program in Biomedical Sciences provides an accelerated track to obtaining both the BS and MD degrees in seven years. Students in the program major in Biomedical Sciences, thus providing extensive background in chemistry, physics, biology, and mathematics, plus exposure to the humanities and social sciences.

In the first three years of the program, students must meet all the requirements of the College of Natural and Agricultural Sciences for a BS degree. Continuation in the program for each student for each of the years is decided by a faculty committee review of academic performance in combination with personal evaluations of each student based on consistent faculty-student contact. Students are required to take the

MCAT during their third year. At the end of the third year at UC-Riverside, selection will be made to identify those individuals who will continue to the medical school phase of the program. Those continuing on to medical school will begin the traditional pre-clinical medical education, but at the UC-Riverside campus. The last two years, which comprise the clinical medical education, will be completed at the UCLA School of Medicine.

Program Title	Thomas Haider Program in Biomedical Sciences
Length of Program	7-years (three undergraduate years).
Number of Students	24
High School Requirements	SAT/ACT, SAT II, GPA/Rank required. (Students enrolled had average SAT of 1327, and GPA of 3.73) Demonstration of maturity and commitment to medicine.
Application Deadline	November 30.
MCAT Requirements	Yes. Minimum scores not defined.

Undergraduate Institution: **University of California—San Diego**
Medical School: University of California—San Diego School of Medicine

Undergraduate Contact Information:	_Medical School Contact Information:_
(same as on right)	Director of Admissions UC – San Diego School of Medicine Office of Admissions 0621 9500 Gilman Drive La Jolla, California 92093 (858) 534-3880
1999-2000 tuition: $9,804	_1999-2000 tuition_: $10,324
http://medschool.ucsd.edu/admissions/med_scholar.html	

About the Medical School:

The School of Medicine is a public institution situated on the main campus of the UC-San Diego. It has an average class size of 120 students.

About the BS-MD Program:

The Medical Scholars Program has been established to encourage the recruitment of unusually talented high school students to promote the goal of increasing diversity at both of the University of California San Diego undergraduate and medical school campuses.

Program Title	The Medical Scholars Program
Length of Program	8-years
Number of Students	12
High School Requirements	Must be a California resident. SAT score of 1450, or ACT score of 32, minimum required. GPA of 4.0, minimum required. Demonstration of strong extra-curricular involvement, particularly in community service and leadership.
Application Deadline	March 24.
MCAT Requirements	None.

Undergraduate Institution: **University of Southern California**
Medical School: University of Southern California Keck
                               School of Medicine

Undergraduate Contact Information:	*Medical School Contact Information:*
Office of Admission	Office of Admissions
College of Letters, Arts, and Sciences	Keck School of Medicine of the
University of Southern California	University of Southern California
Los Angeles, CA 90089	1975 Zonal Avenue (KAM 100-C)
(213) 740-5930	Los Angeles, CA 90033
cas@mizar.usc.edu	(323) 442-2552
1999-2000 tuition: $22,200	*1999-2000 tuition*: $32,266
http://www.usc.edu/schools/medicine/	

About the Medical School:

The University of Southern California is a private, non-denominational, co-educational university. The School of Medicine was established in 1885 and is situated across from its chief teaching hospital, the Los Angeles County/USC Medical Center. The average class size is 150 students.

About the BA/BS-MD Program:

The program was initiated in 1993 in the hope to encourage highly motivated students to expand the breadth of their education through a diverse liberal arts education beyond the standard premedical curriculum. The goal is to produce physicians who are educated in medical science as well as the arts and humanities.

The program is unaccelerated and students may pursue any major offered by the university that is compatible with the requirements of the program. Advancement to the medical school is based on acceptable academic performance and MCAT scores, as defined by the program.

Program Title	The Baccalaureate/MD Program
Length of Program	8-years
Number of Students	20
High School Requirements	No specific SAT/ACT or GPA requirements. (Students enrolled had average SAT of 1500 and GPA of 4.2) Demonstration of leadership and community involvement.
Application Deadline	November 15.
MCAT Requirements	Yes. Minimum scores not defined.

Undergraduate Institution: **University of Connecticut**
Medical School: University of Connecticut School of Medicine

Undergraduate Contact Information:	*Medical School Contact Information:*
Office of Admissions	Admissions Center
University of Connecticut	University of Connecticut School of Medicine
Storrs, CT 06269	263 Farmington Avenue, Rm. AG-062
(860) 486-2000	Farmington, CT 06030
premed@oracle.pnb.uconn.edu	(860) 679-4713
1999-2000 tuition: $5,398 ($13,916 for non-residents)	*1999-2000 tuition*: $9,375 ($21,320 for non-residents)
http://www.ucc.uconn.edu/~beahusky/combmed.html	

About the Medical School:

The University of Connecticut School of Medicine is a public institution established in 1968. The average class size is 80 students.

About the BS-MD Program:

This program offers gifted and talented high school students who are focused on a career in medicine the opportunity to combine a broad-based liberal arts program with their medical education.

Program Title	Combined Program in Medicine
Length of Program	8-years.
Number of Students	
High School Requirements	Preference is given to Connecticut residents. SAT score of 1300, or ACT score of 30, minimum required. GPA of 3.5 / 4.0, minimum required. High School rank within top 5%.
Application Deadline	January 1.
MCAT Requirements	Yes. Minimum scores not defined.

Undergraduate Institution: **George Washington University (7-Year)**
Medical School: George Washington University School of
                               Medicine

Undergraduate Contact Information:	*Medical School Contact Information:*
Office of Admissions	Office of Admissions
George Washington University	George Washington University School of Medicine
2121 "I" Street, NW	Room 716
Washington, DC 20052	2300 Eye Street, NW
(800) 447-3765	Washington, DC 20037
	(202) 994-3506
1999-2000 tuition: $30,500	*1999-2000 tuition*: $30,500
http://www.gwumc.edu/smhs/	

About the Medical School:

The George Washington School of Medicine is a private institution that opened in 1825. The school of medicine is situated near the main GW campus in downtown Washington, DC. The average class size is 150 students.

About the BA-MD Program:

The 7-year BA/MD Program was initiated to provide premedical students the opportunity to explore other fields of interest. The course requirements for the baccalaureate degree in the humanities and social sciences vary, but students must complete 32 semester hours in the natural and physical sciences. Accepted students are required to take the MCAT, but it will not be used as a factor for promotion. Students will receive their baccalaureate degree after completion of the first year of medical school.

Program Title	The 7-Year BA/MD Program
Length of Program	7-years (three undergraduate years).
Number of Students	10
High School Requirements	SAT scores of 650 math and 710 verbal, minimum required. Or, ACT score of 32, minimum required. SAT II required in writing, math, and a science. GPA of at least 3.7 / 4.0, minimum required. High School rank within the top 5%.
Application Deadline	December 1.
MCAT Requirements	Yes. Minimum scores not defined.

Undergraduate Institution: **George Washington University (8-Year)**
Medical School: George Washington University School of
                               Medicine

Undergraduate Contact Information:	*Medical School Contact Information:*
Office of Admissions	Office of Admissions, Room 716
George Washington University	George Washington University School of Medicine
2121 "I" Street, NW	2300 Eye Street, NW
Washington, DC 20052	Washington, DC 20037
(800) 447-3765	(202) 994-3506
1999-2000 tuition: $30,500	*1999-2000 tuition:* $30,500
http://www.gwumc.edu/smhs/	

About the Medical School:

The George Washington School of Medicine is a private institution that opened in 1825. The school of medicine is situated near the main GW campus in downtown Washington, DC. The average class size is 150 students.

About the BA-MD Program:

This program is for highly qualified high school students who are interested in pursuing an engineering or computer science degree and then an MD degree. This program is an unaccelerated and unabridged 8-year course with accepted students spending the first four years in the School of Engineering and Applied Science and the next four years in the GW School of Medicine and Health Sciences.

Program Title	Integrated Engineering and Medicine Program
Length of Program	8-years.
Number of Students	
High School Requirements	SAT scores of 650 math and 710 verbal, minimum required. Or, ACT score of 32, minimum required. SAT II required in writing, math, and a science. GPA of at least 3.7 / 4.0, minimum required. High School rank within the top 5%.
Application Deadline	December 1.
MCAT Requirements	Yes. Minimum scores not defined.

Undergraduate Institution: **Howard University**
Medical School: Howard University College of Medicine

Undergraduate Contact Information:	*Medical School Contact Information:*
Center for Pre-Professional Education	Office of Admissions
PO Box 473	Howard University College of Medicine
Administrative Building	520 W Street, NW
Washington, DC 20059	Washington, DC 20059
(202) 806-7231	(202) 806-6270
1999-2000 tuition: $9,390	*1999-2000 tuition*: $16,950

About the Medical School:

The Howard University College of Medicine is a private institution and is the oldest and largest historically black medical school in the country. It opened in 1868. The College's goal is to train students to become competent, compassionate physicians who will provide care in medically underserved communities. The average class size is 110 students.

About the BA/BS-MD Program:

The goal of this accelerated combined-degree is to encourage talented undergraduate students to choose medicine as a career and to retain these students at the Howard University College of Medicine. The program leads to a bachelor's degree awarded by the College of Arts and Sciences and the MD degree by the College of Medicine. Students must complete 40 semester hours of humanities and social sciences and at least 46 semester hours of natural and physical sciences within two years. The MCAT is also required and is to be taken in the spring of the second year. Progression to the medical school is contingent upon the results of the MCAT and GPA.

Program Title	6-Year Combined Degree Program.
Length of Program	6-years (two undergraduate years).
Number of Students	10
High School Requirements	High School rank within top 5%. No specific SAT or ACT requirements. (Students enrolled had average SAT of 1300 and GPA of 3.7)
Application Deadline	Rolling
MCAT Requirements	Yes. Minimum scores not defined.

Undergraduate Institution: **University of Florida**
Medical School: University of Florida College of
                               Medicine

Undergraduate Contact Information:	_Medical School Contact Information:_
(same as on right)	Medical Selection Committee University of Florida College of medicine PO Box 100216 Gainesville, FL 32610 (352) 392-4569
1999-2000 tuition: $1,480 ($8,136 for non-residents)	_1999-2000 tuition_: $9,684 ($27,335 for non-residents)

About the Medical School:

The University of Florida College of Medicine is a public institution opened in 1956. It is situated in the University of Florida main campus and is a component of the University of Florida Health Science Center. The average class size is 75 students.

About the BS-MD Program:

The Junior Honors Medical Program is designed for undergraduate students who have chosen a career in the medical profession and who have demonstrated superior scholastic ability and personal development during the first two years of their undergraduate studies. Students are selected during their sophomore year at the University of Florida in Gainesville. Selection is based on sophomore standing, GPA, prerequisite courses, and SAT scores. The MCAT is required but not a factor for admission to the medical school.

Program Title	The Junior Honors Medical Program
Length of Program	8-years
Number of Students	12
High School Requirements	Must be a sophomore at the University of Florida. SAT is required.
Application Deadline	January 31.
MCAT Requirements	Yes. Minimum scores not defined.

Undergraduate Institution: **University of Miami (6-year)**
Medical School: University of Miami School of Medicine

Undergraduate Contact Information:	*Medical School Contact Information:*
Office of Admissions	Office of Admissions
University of Miami	University of Miami School of Medicine
PO Box 248025	PO Box 016159
Coral Gables, FL 33124	Miami, FL 33101
(305) 284-4323	(305) 243-6791
1999-2000 tuition: $21,350	*1999-2000 tuition*: $25,670
http://www.miami.edu/medical-admissions	

About the Medical School:

The University of Miami School of Medicine is a private institution and is the largest and oldest medical school in Florida. It was founded in 1952. The School of Medicine is located on the medical campus next to Jackson Memorial Hospital in the Civic Center area of Miami. The average class size is 140 students.

About the BS-MD Program:

The Honors Program in Medicine is the University of Miami's 6-year BS/MD program. It was established in 1981 and is operated by the School of Medicine in conjunction with the School of Arts and Sciences. It offers exceptionally motivated and talented students who have reached a mature decision to study medicine based on their experiences an opportunity to earn the BS and MD degrees in either 6 or 7 years.

The first two or three years are spent on the Coral Gables campus of the University of Miami taking the required courses for their major. Students must maintain a minimum cumulative GPA of 3.4, and a minimum science GPA of 3.2. Students must also take the MCAT before starting medical school. The MCAT score is not required for promotion but to assess the student's level of preparedness. The Baccalaureate degree is received following the first year of medical studies.

Program Title	
	The Honors Program in Medicine
Length of Program	6 or 7-years (two or three undergraduate years).
Number of Students	20
High School Requirements	Must be a Florida resident. SAT score of 1360, or ACT score of 31, minimum required. SAT II subject tests in English, Mathematics, and one Science.
Application Deadline	January 15.
MCAT Requirements	Yes. Minimum scores not defined.

Undergraduate Institution: **University of Miami** (7-year)
Medical School: University of Miami School of Medicine

Undergraduate Contact Information:	_Medical School Contact Information:_
Office of Admissions	Office of Admissions
PO Box 24805	University of Miami School of Medicine
Coral Gables, FL 33124	PO Box 016159
(305) 284-4323	Miami, FL 33101
	(305) 243-6791
1999-2000 tuition: $21,350	_1999-2000 tuition_: $25,670
http://www.miami.edu/medical-admissions	

About the Medical School:

   The University of Miami School of Medicine is a private institution and is the largest and oldest medical school in Florida. It was founded in 1952. The School of Medicine is located on the medical campus next to Jackson Memorial Hospital in the Civic Center area of Miami. The average class size is 140 students.

About the BS-MD Program:

   The Medical Scholars Program accepts exceptionally capable students at the end of their sophomore year at the University of Miami. With admission into the program, students are assured a place in the freshman class of the School of Medicine after successfully completing the program requirements, which includes completion of the junior year of undergraduate studies at the University of Miami. Following the junior year and the completion of 90 credits, students begin their medical studies at the School of Medicine. To be promoted, students must maintain a cumulative GPA of 3.4 and a science GPA of 3.2. Upon successful completion of the first year of medical studies, students will be granted their appropriate bachelor's degrees.

Program Title	The Medical Scholars Program
Length of Program	7-years (three undergraduate years).
Number of Students	
High School Requirements	Must be a Florida resident. Must complete freshman year with a GPA of 3.4. SAT score of 1270, or ACT score of 29, minimum required.
Application Deadline	March 15 of freshman year.
MCAT Requirements	None.

Undergraduate Institution: **Illinois Institute of Technology**
Medical School: Finch University of the Health
                            Sciences—Chicago Medical School

Undergraduate Contact Information:	_Medical School Contact Information:_
Dean of Admission	Office of Admissions
BS/MD Program	Chicago Medical School
Illinois Institute of Technology	3333 Green Bay Road
10 West 33rd Street	Chicago, IL 60064
Chicago, IL 60616	(847) 578-3206
(312) 567-3025	
admissions@vax1.ais.iit.edu	
1999-2000 tuition: $17,500	_1999-2000 tuition:_ $33,527
http://www.iit.edu/~premed/index.html	

About the Medical School:

The Chicago Medical School is a private institution founded in 1912 as a part of the Finch University of Health Sciences, situated in North Chicago. The average class size is 165 students.

About the BS-MD Program:

The Honors Program in Engineering and Medicine is designed to allow students to earn both a Bachelor of Science degree in chemical, computer, electrical, mechanical engineering, molecular biochemistry and biophysics, or computer science, as well as an MD degree in eight years. The goal is to produce graduates who understand the intricacies of technology applied to medicine who will be the future innovators in improving medical diagnoses and treatment for their patients.

The curriculum focuses on studies for the bachelor's degree in the first four years. Continuation on to medical school is contingent upon maintaining a 3.3 GPA. No course grade below a "C" is allowed.

Program Title	Honors Program in Engineering and Medicine
Length of Program	8-years.
Number of Students	15
High School Requirements	No specific SAT/ACT or GPA requirements. (Students enrolled had average SAT of 1350 and GPA of 4.0) Demonstration of interest in engineering and medicine.
Application Deadline	January 15.
MCAT Requirements	None.

Undergraduate Institution: **Illinois Institute of Technology**
Medical School: Rush Medical College

Undergraduate Contact Information:	_Medical School Contact Information:_
Dean of Admission	Office of Admissions
Illinois Institute of Technology	524 Armour Academic Center
BS/MD Program	Rush Medical College
10 West 33rd Street	600 South Paulina Avenue
Chicago, IL 60616	Chicago, IL 60612
(312) 567-3025	(312) 942-6913
admissions@vax1.ais.iit.edu	
1999-2000 tuition: $17,500	_1999-2000 tuition_: $27,120
http://www.iit.edu/~premed/index.html	

About the Medical School:

Rush Medical College is a private institution founded in 1837 and is the oldest component of Rush University. The original medical college closed in 1942, but then reopened in 1971. The Rush Medical College is affiliated with multiple hospitals and a neighborhood health center, the Rush-Presbyterian-St Luke's Medical Center. The average class size is 120 students.

About the BS-MD Program:

The IIT/Rush Medical College combined program is a six-year program open to current IIT sophomores. Students admitted to this program will complete their undergraduate degree at IIT either in chemical engineering, mechanical engineering, electrical engineering, computer science, or molecular biochemistry & biophysics during the first two years of the program. As part of this experience they will participate in a two-semester research project that bridges engineering, science, and medicine. The final four years of the program are spent at Rush Medical

College. This program is designed for students who intend to become research-oriented physicians.

Program Title	Honors Program in Engineering and Medicine
Length of Program	8-years.
Number of Students	
High School Requirements	Must be a sophomore at the Illinois Institute of Technology. Demonstration of interest in engineering and medicine.
Application Deadline	December 1 of sophomore year.
MCAT Requirements	None.

Undergraduate Institution: **Northwestern University**
Medical School: Northwestern University Medical School

Undergraduate Contact Information:	*Medical School Contact Information:*
Office of Admission and Finacial Aid	Northwestern University Medical School
PO Box 3060	303 East Chicago Avenue
1801 Hinman Avenue	Chicago, IL 60611
Evanston, IL 60204	(312) 503-8206
(708) 491-7271	
ug-admissions@nwu.edu	
1999-2000 tuition: $23,562	*1999-2000 tuition*: $30,417
http://www.nums.nwu.edu/viewbook/bamdprog.htm	

About the Medical School:

Northwestern University Medical School is a private institution founded in 1859. The medical campus is situated at Northwestern University's lakefront Chicago campus. The medical students gain their clinical experience at the McGaw Hospitals, which is a group of urban, suburban, specialized, and general hospitals throughout the Chicago area. The average class size is 165 students.

About the BA/BS-MD Program:

Northwestern's Honors Program in Medical Education accelerates the premedical phase of study so that the MD degree may be obtained seven years after entry into the University. The first three years of the program are spent on the Evanston campus and the last four at the Medical School on the lakefront Chicago campus. A student may choose one of several options to complete undergraduate preparation in medicine. In the Weinberg College of Arts and Sciences, the student may pursue an honors-level concentration in a specific department. The School of Speech offers students an opportunity to study communication sciences.

Also, students may major in biomedical engineering in the McCormick School of Engineering and Applied Science.

Program Title	The BA/MD Honors Program in Medical Education
Length of Program	7-years (three undergraduate years)
Number of Students	40
High School Requirements	The SAT or ACT required. The SAT II (in mathematics IIC, chemistry, writing) required. (Students enrolled had average SAT over 1500 and SAT II scores of 768 mathematics, 750 chemistry, and 763 writing) Demonstration of motivation, concern for others, and maturity.
Application Deadline	January 1.
MCAT Requirements	None.

Undergraduate Institution: **University of Illinois at Chicago**
Medical School: University of Illinois at Chicago College
                               of Medicine

Undergraduate Contact Information:	*Medical School Contact Information:*
Special Projects Unit	Medical College Admissions
Office of Admissions and Records	Room 165 CME M/C 783
University of Illinois at Chicago	UIC College of Medicine
PO Box 6020	808 South Wood Street
Chicago, IL 60680	Chicago, IL 60612
(312) 996-8365	(312) 996-5635
1999-2000 tuition: $3,138	*1999-2000 tuition*: $16,294
($9,414 for non-residents)	($39,826 for non-residents)
http://www.uic.edu/depts/oaa/spec_prog/gppa/	

About the Medical School:

The UIC College of Medicine is a public institution originally founded as the College of Physicians and Surgeons of Chicago in 1881. The institution changed its name to the University of Illinois College of Medicine in 1900. The average class size is 300 students.

About the BS-MD Program:

The Guaranteed Professional Program Admission to the College of Medicine is part of UIC's larger program to admit motivated and highly qualified freshmen annually to UIC with admission guaranteed, if criteria are met, to one of their professional degree programs. The goal is to allow students to focus on their undergraduate studies and have the opportunity to become well rounded and educated in multiple areas before pursuing their professional studies.

The specific goal of the Guaranteed Professional Program Admission to the College of Medicine is to encourage motivated students to choose medicine as a career and to enter the UIC College of Medicine for their medical education. Accepted students must enroll in the Honors College and complete their baccalaureate requirements within three to five years. Students must maintain a GPA of 4.5 (out of 5.0) and take the MCAT during their junior year.

Program Title	The Guaranteed Professional Program Admissions to the **College of Medicine**
Length of Program	8-years.
Number of Students	60
High School Requirements	Must be an Illinois resident. SAT score of 1240 or ACT score of 28, minimum required. High School rank in the top 15%, minimum required.
Application Deadline	January 15.
MCAT Requirements	Yes. Not a factor for promotion to medical school.

Undergraduate Institution: **Indiana State University**
Medical School: Indiana University School of Medicine

Undergraduate Contact Information:	_Medical School Contact Information:_
Associate Dean,	Medical School Admissions Office
College of Arts and Sciences	Fesler Hall 213
Indiana State University	Indiana University School of Medicine
Terre Haute, IN 47809	1120 South Drive
(812) 237-2781	Indianapolis, IN 46202
	(317) 274-3772
1999-2000 tuition: $1,782	_1999-2000 tuition_: $13,245
http://www.medicine.iu.edu/admpage.html	

About the Medical School:

The Indiana University School of Medicine is a public institution founded in 1903. It is the only medical school in the state. The school has multiple campuses throughout Indiana where students can spend the first two years of medical school. The average class size is 280 students.

About the BA-MD Program:

The BA/MD Rural Health Program is designed to address the rural health needs of the State of Indiana by providing increased opportunities for residents from rural communities to obtain education and training in medicine. During the undergraduate component of the program students enrolled in the rural health program will participate in special experiences designed to enhance their careers as medical practitioners in rural settings. The curriculum will be a traditional premed curriculum that has been modified to enhance the likelihood of success in the practice of rural medicine.

Admissions into the program will be limited to Indiana residents from rural communities. Accepted students are required to maintain a minimum cumulative GPA of 3.5 and take the MCAT for promotion to the medical school.

Program Title	BA/MD Rural Health Program
Length of Program	8-years.
Number of Students	10
High School Requirements	Must be an Indiana resident. SAT score of 1200 or ACT score of 27, minimum required. GPA of 3.5 / 4.0, minimum required. Must have lived in a federally designated area that is not metropolitan or is designated as a rural census tract.
Application Deadline	December 1.
MCAT Requirements	Yes. Must achieve a score equal to the mean of the previous year's matriculating class.

Undergraduate Institution: **Boston University**
Medical School: Boston University School of Medicine

Undergraduate Contact Information:	_Medical School Contact Information:_
Office of Admissions	Admissions Office
121 Bay State Road	Boston University School of Medicine
Boston, MA 02215	715 Albany Street
(617) 353-2300	Boston, MA 02118
admissions@bu.edu	(617) 638-4630
1999-2000 tuition: $23,770	_1999-2000 tuition_: $35,525
http://web.bu.edu/admissions/academics/esp/la/index.html	

About the Medical School:

The Boston University School of Medicine is a private institution founded in 1873 by Boston University at the site of the original New England Female Medical College. The School of Medicine is part of the larger Boston Medical Center. The average class size is 150 students.

About the BA-MD Program:

The Seven-Year Liberal Arts/Medical Education Program integrates the undergraduate and medical school curriculum, thereby shortening the overall period of study. Students who are accepted into the program are admitted to the College of Arts and Sciences, and provisionally to Boston University School of Medicine. The combined curriculum offers extensive elective options for study in the humanities and social sciences. The flexible nature of the program allows students to develop their academic interests while fulfilling premedical requirements at an accelerated and more rigorous level. Students receive their Bachelor of Arts degree in Medical Science at the completion of the fourth year (which constitutes their first full year of medical study as graduate students), and the Doctor of Medicine degree at the completion of the seventh year. Students must maintain a minimum overall GPA of 3.2 and take the MCAT during the spring of their second year.

Program Title	The Seven-Year Liberal Arts/Medical Education Program
Length of Program	7-years (three undergraduate years).
Number of Students	20
High School Requirements	The SAT or ACT, and Rank required. The SAT II (in writing, mathematics, and chemistry) required. (Students enrolled had average SAT over 1500, SAT II subject scores of 750, GPA of 3.94/4.00, and high school in top 1%). Demonstration of motivation, maturity, and understanding of a career in medicine.
Application Deadline	December 1.
MCAT Requirements	Yes. Minimum score of 28 required.

Undergraduate Institution: **Boston University**
Medical School: UMDNJ—New Jersey Medical School

Undergraduate Contact Information:	_Medical School Contact Information:_
Office of Admissions	Office of Admissions
Boston University	C653 MSB
121 Bay State Road	UMDNJ – New Jersey Medical School
Boston, MA 02215	185 South Orange Avenue
(617) 353-2300	Newark, NJ 07103
admissions@bu.edu	(973) 972-4631
1999-2000 tuition: $23,770	_1999-2000 tuition_: $16,052
http://web.bu.edu/admissions/academics/esp/la/njres.html	

About the Medical School:

The New Jersey Medical School of the University of Medicine and Dentistry of New Jersey is a public institution established in Newark, New Jersey in 1977. The average medical school class size is 170 students.

The New Jersey Medical School has established accelerated baccalaureate/MD-degree programs in collaboration with different undergraduate institutions. The goal of these programs is to give highly qualified high school students an opportunity to broaden their premedical preparation without having to compete for admission to medical school.

About the BA-MD Program:

Boston University College of Arts and Sciences and UMDNJ-New Jersey Medical School offers New Jersey residents the opportunity to participate in an accelerated education that leads to the Bachelor of Arts degree from Boston University and the Doctor of Medicine degree from the New Jersey Medical School. Students admitted to the program spend three years and one summer term at the Boston University College of Arts and Sciences, and one summer of biomedical research at the New Jersey Medical School. At the beginning of the fourth academic year, students enter UMDNJ and pursue the traditional four-year medical school curriculum. The baccalaureate degree will be granted following completion of the first year of medical school.

Accepted students must maintain a minimum GPA of 3.4 during their three years of undergraduate studies. Students must take the MCAT, but will not be a factor for promotion or admission to the medical school.

Program Title	The 7-Year Liberal Arts / UMDNJ Medical Program
Length of Program	7-years (three undergraduate years)
Number of Students	No quota.
High School Requirements	Must be a New Jersey resident. SAT score of 1400, minimum required. High School rank in the top 10%, minimum required.
Application Deadline	January 7.
MCAT Requirements	Yes. Not a factor for promotion to medical school.

Undergraduate Institution: **Michigan State University**
Medical School: Michigan State University College of
                            Human Medicine

Undergraduate Contact Information:	*Medical School Contact Information:*
College of Human Medicine	Office of Admissions
Office of Admissions	College of Human Medicine
A-239 Life Sciences	A-239 Life Sciences
East Lansing, MI 48824	Michigan State University
(517) 353-9620	East Lansing, MI 48824
	(517) 353-9620
1999-2000 tuition: $4,670	*1999-2000 tuition*: $15,423
($12,034 for non-residents)	($33,873 for non-residents)
http://www.chm.msu.edu/chmhome/admissn.htm	

About the Medical School:

The College of Human Medicine is a public institution founded in 1964 in response to Michigan's growing need for primary care physicians. The medical school is situated on the main campus of Michigan State University. Students are taught at the main campus at East Lansing for the first two years. Afterwards, students are sent to one of six community campuses for their clinical training. The average class size is 106.

About the BA/BS-MD Program:

The College of Human Medicine Medical Scholars Program offers a unique enrichment opportunity for academically talented freshmen. Successful applicants for this program are high achieving high school seniors who demonstrate their interest in becoming physicians through medical/clinical experiences and community leadership experiences.

Accepted students are expected to fulfill all of the Baccalaureate degree requirements within 3 to 5 years, the College of Human Medicine pre-medical requirements, and the Medical Scholars

Academic 3 Components requirements. Students must maintain a minimal cumulative GPA of 3.2, and a minimum premedical courses GPA of 3.0.

Program Title	The Medical Scholars Program
Length of Program	8-years.
Number of Students	10
High School Requirements	Preference is given to Michigan residents. Demonstration of strong interest in becoming physicians through clinical experiences and community leadership experiences.
Application Deadline	November 1.
MCAT Requirements	None.

Undergraduate Institution: **University of Michigan**
Medical School: University of Michigan Medical School

Undergraduate Contact Information:	*Medical School Contact Information:*
Inteflex Program	Admissions Office
3808 Medical Science Building II	M4130 Medical Science I Building
1301 Catherine Street	University of Michigan Medical School
Ann Arbor, MI 48109	Ann Arbor, MI 48109
(734) 763-3265	(734) 764-6317
alburdi@umich.edu	
1999-2000 tuition: $7,468 ($23,790 for non-residents)	*1999-2000 tuition*: $18,020 ($27,776 for non-residents)
http://www.med.umich.edu/medschool/inteflex/	

About the Medical School:

The University of Michigan Medical School is a public institution founded in 1850. The average class size is 170 students.

About the BS-MD Program:

The Inteflex Program is short for the University of Michigan's Integrated Premedical/Medical BS/MD-Program. The program's goal is to educate physicians who are scientifically competent, compassionate, and socially conscious and who can apply the insights gained in the study of the humanities and social sciences in addressing the challenges of medicine in the twenty-first century.

At the time of this writing, this program was currently on hold and under review. Please contact the Inteflex Program at the above contact information for further details.

Program Title	The Inteflex Program
Length of Program	8-years.
Number of Students	35
High School Requirements	SAT score of 1310, or ACT score of 29, minimum required. (Students enrolled had average SAT over 1400, GPA of 3.94)
Application Deadline	N/A
MCAT Requirements	Yes. Minimum score not defined.

Undergraduate Institution: **University of Missouri—Kansas City**
Medical School: University of Missouri—Kansas City School of Medicine

Undergraduate Contact Information: (same as on right)	*Medical School Contact Information:* Council on Selection UMKC School of Medicine 2411 Holmes Kansas City, MO 64108 (816) 235-1870
1999-2000 tuition: $19,948 ($40,250 for non-residents)	*1999-2000 tuition*: $21,322 ($43,200 for non-residents)
http://research.med.umkc.edu/	

About the Medical School:

The University of Missouri—Kansas City School of Medicine is a public institution founded in 1969. Located on suburban Hospital Hill campus, the medical school is near both the schools and colleges of the university and affiliated hospitals. The School of Medicine, in combination with the College of Arts and Sciences and the School of Biological Sciences, offers a year-round program leading to baccalaureate and MD degrees in six years. The average class size is 100 students.

About the BA/BS-MD Program:

The University of Missouri—Kansas City School of Medicine's primary educational mission is a combined baccalaureate/doctor of medicine degree program directly out of high school. It is an integrated program with a mix of liberal arts, basic medical sciences, and clinical medicine throughout the curriculum. The program has ongoing clinical involvement that begins from the first year and progressively increases. The program features an eleven-month curriculum with a one-month vacation, and structures academic and clinical experiences to provide both degrees in six years from the same institution. You apply only once, initially. Students spend three-quarters of their time the first two years working towards their baccalaureate requirements. Conversely, students spend three-quarters of their last four years completing their MD requirements. Thereby, the study of medicine and liberal arts are integrated for all six years.

Program Title	The School of Medicine Six-Year Program
Length of Program	6-years (integrated baccalaureate and medical curriculum).
Number of Students	120
High School Requirements	ACT score and GPA are required. Minimums not defined. (Students enrolled had average ACT scores in the 90th percentile) Demonstration of maturity, leadership, stamina, motivation for medicine, and job experience.
Application Deadline	November 15.
MCAT Requirements	None.

Undergraduate Institution: **The College of New Jersey**
Medical School: UMDNJ—New Jersey Medical School

Undergraduate Contact Information:	*Medical School Contact Information:*
Medical Careers Committee	Office of Admissions
The College of New Jersey	C653 MSB
PO Box 7718	UMDNJ – New Jersey Medical School
Ewing, NJ 08628	185 South Orange Avenue
(609) 771-2021	Newark, NJ 07103
medcar@tcnj.edu	(973) 972-4631
1999-2000 tuition: $5,685 ($9,002 for non-residents)	*1999-2000 tuition*: $16,052 ($25,119 for non-residents)
http://www.tcnj.edu/prospective/ac_prog/	

About the Medical School:

The New Jersey Medical School of the University of Medicine and Dentistry of New Jersey is a public institution established in Newark, New Jersey in 1977. The average medical school class size is 170 students.

The New Jersey Medical School has established accelerated baccalaureate/MD-degree programs in collaboration with different undergraduate institutions. The goal of these programs is to give highly qualified high school students an opportunity to broaden their premedical preparation without having to compete for admission to medical school.

About the BS-MD Program:

As a participant in the program, students must maintain an overall minimum GPA of 3.4, and maintain a minimum science GPA of 3.4. Also, students must engage in research at the New Jersey Medical School over a summer during their undergraduate studies. Finally, although no minimum score is required on the test, students must also sit for the MCAT.

Program Title	The 7-Year Combined BS/MD Program
Length of Program	7-years (three years of undergraduate)
Number of Students	No quota.
High School Requirements	SAT score of 1400, minimum required. High School rank in the top 10%, minimum required.
Application Deadline	January 7.
MCAT Requirements	Yes. Not a factor for promotion to medical school.

Undergraduate Institution: **Drew University**
Medical School: UMDNJ—New Jersey Medical School

Undergraduate Contact Information:	*Medical School Contact Information:*
College of Admissions Drew University Madison, NJ 07940 (973) 408-3739 cadm@drew.edu	Office of Admissions C653 MSB UMDNJ – New Jersey Medical School 185 South Orange Avenue Newark, NJ 07103 (973) 972-4631
1999-2000 tuition: $25,503	*1999-2000 tuition*: $16,052 ($25,119 for non-residents)
http://www.drew.edu/cla/depts/programs/dual-degree-med.html	

About the Medical School:

The New Jersey Medical School of the University of Medicine and Dentistry of New Jersey is a public institution established in Newark, New Jersey in 1977. The average medical school class size is 170 students.

The New Jersey Medical School has established accelerated baccalaureate/MD-degree programs in collaboration with different undergraduate institutions. The goal of these programs is to give highly qualified high school students an opportunity to broaden their premedical preparation without having to compete for admission to medical school.

About the BA-MD Program:

The College of Liberal Arts of Drew University sponsors this program where students in the program may major in any area, except Arts and Behavioral Sciences. The required pre-medical courses must be completed within the three-year period at Drew, in addition to the requirements of the selected major and the general education requirements for the liberal arts degree.

Students must maintain an overall minimum GPA of 3.4 each semester. In addition, students must maintain a minimum science GPA of 3.4 each semester at Drew, with a minimum of B- in each of the required pre-medical courses. Finally, although no minimum score is required on the test for candidates who have remained in good academic standing, students must also sit for the MCAT during their junior year.

Program Title	The Dual Degree Medical Program
Length of Program	7-years (three undergraduate years).
Number of Students	No quota.
High School Requirements	SAT score of 1400, minimum required. High School rank in the top 10%, minimum required.
Application Deadline	January 7.
MCAT Requirements	Yes. Not a factor for promotion to medical school.

Undergraduate Institution: **Montclair State University**
Medical School: UMDNJ—New Jersey Medical School

Undergraduate Contact Information:	_Medical School Contact Information:_
Health Professions Committee	Office of Admissions
Department of Biology	C653 MSB
Montclair State University	UMDNJ – New Jersey Medical School
Upper Montclair, NJ 07043	185 South Orange Avenue
(973) 655-5116	Newark, NJ 07103
	(973) 972-4631
1999-2000 tuition: $4,320	_1999-2000 tuition_: $16,052
($6,235 for non-residents)	($25,119 for non-residents)

About the Medical School:

The New Jersey Medical School of the University of Medicine and Dentistry of New Jersey is a public institution established in Newark, New Jersey in 1977. The average medical school class size is 170 students.

The New Jersey Medical School has established accelerated baccalaureate/MD-degree programs in collaboration with different undergraduate institutions. The goal of these programs is to give highly qualified high school students an opportunity to broaden their premedical preparation without having to compete for admission to medical school.

About the BS-MD Program:

As a participant in the program, students must maintain an overall minimum GPA of 3.4, and maintain a minimum science GPA of 3.4. Also, students must engage in research at the New Jersey Medical School over a summer during their undergraduate studies. Finally, although no minimum score is required on the test, students must also sit for the MCAT.

Program Title	The 7-Year BS/MD Program
Length of Program	7-years (three undergraduate years)
Number of Students	No quota.
High School Requirements	SAT score of 1400, minimum required. High School rank in the top 10%, minimum required.
Application Deadline	January 7.
MCAT Requirements	Yes. Not a factor for promotion to medical school.

Undergraduate Institution: **New Jersey Institute of Technology**
Medical School: UMDNJ—New Jersey Medical School

Undergraduate Contact Information:	_Medical School Contact Information:_
Honors College New Jersey Institute of Technology University Heights, Newark, NJ 07102 (973) 596-3216 honors@njit.edu	Office of Admissions C653 MSB UMDNJ – New Jersey Medical School 185 South Orange Avenue Newark, NJ 07103 (973) 972-4631
1999-2000 tuition: $6,480 ($10,824 for non-residents)	_1999-2000 tuition_: $16,052 ($25,119 for non-residents)
http://www.njit.edu/esc/	

About the Medical School:

The New Jersey Medical School of the University of Medicine and Dentistry of New Jersey is a public institution established in Newark, New Jersey in 1977. The average medical school class size is 170 students.

The New Jersey Medical School has established accelerated baccalaureate/MD-degree programs in collaboration with different undergraduate institutions. The goal of these programs is to give highly qualified high school students an opportunity to broaden their premedical preparation without having to compete for admission to medical school.

About the BS-MD Program:

The BS/MD Program is an accelerated seven-year program in premedicine. In the accelerated seven-year program, students study for three years at NJIT, followed by the traditional four years at the UMDNJ—New Jersey Medical School. Students are awarded a bachelors degree in Engineering Science upon the successful completion of their first year of professional studies at the New Jersey Medical School.

As a participant in the program, students must maintain an overall minimum GPA of 3.4, and maintain a minimum science GPA of 3.4. Also, students must engage in research at the New Jersey Medical School over a summer during their undergraduate studies. Finally, although no minimum score is required on the test, students must also sit for the MCAT.

Program Title	The 7-Year Accelerated BS/MD Program
Length of Program	7-years (three undergraduate years)
Number of Students	No quota.
High School Requirements	SAT score of 1400, minimum required. High School rank in the top 10%, minimum required.
Application Deadline	January 7.
MCAT Requirements	Yes. Not a factor for promotion to medical school.

Undergraduate Institution: **Richard Stockton College of New Jersey**
Medical School: UMDNJ—New Jersey Medical School

Undergraduate Contact Information:	_Medical School Contact Information:_
Office of the Associate Vice President, Academic Affairs Stockton State College Pomona, NJ 08240 (609) 652-4514 admissions@stockton.edu	Office of Admissions C653 MSB UMDNJ – New Jersey Medical School 185 South Orange Avenue Newark, NJ 07103 (973) 972-4631
1999-2000 tuition: $4,400 ($6,432 for non-residents)	_1999-2000 tuition_: $16,052 ($25,119 for non-residents)

About the Medical School:

The New Jersey Medical School of the University of Medicine and Dentistry of New Jersey is a public institution established in Newark, New Jersey in 1977. The average medical school class size is 170 students.

The New Jersey Medical School has established accelerated baccalaureate/MD-degree programs in collaboration with different undergraduate institutions. The goal of these programs is to give highly qualified high school students an opportunity to broaden their premedical preparation without having to compete for admission to medical school.

About the BS-MD Program:

As a participant in the program, students must maintain an overall minimum GPA of 3.4, and maintain a minimum science GPA of 3.4. Also, students must engage in research at the New Jersey Medical School over a summer during their undergraduate studies. Finally, although no minimum score is required on the test, students must also sit for the MCAT.

Program Title	The 7-Year BS/MD Program
Length of Program	7-years (three undergraduate years)
Number of Students	No quota.
High School Requirements	SAT score of 1400, minimum required. High School rank in the top 10%, minimum required.
Application Deadline	January 7.
MCAT Requirements	Yes. Not a factor for promotion to medical school.

Undergraduate Institution: **Rutgers University—Newark Campus**
Medical School: UMDNJ—New Jersey Medical School

Undergraduate Contact Information:	_Medical School Contact Information:_
Office of Admissions	Office of Admissions
Rutgers University	C653 MSB
249 University Avenue	UMDNJ – New Jersey Medical School
Newark, NJ	185 South Orange Avenue
(973) 353-5205	Newark, NJ 07103
	(973) 972-4631
1999-2000 tuition: $4,762	_1999-2000 tuition_: $16,052
($9,962 for non-residents)	($25,119 for non-residents)
http://lifesci.rutgers.edu/~hpo	

About the Medical School:

The New Jersey Medical School of the University of Medicine and Dentistry of New Jersey is a public institution established in Newark, New Jersey in 1977. The average medical school class size is 170 students.

The New Jersey Medical School has established accelerated baccalaureate/MD-degree programs in collaboration with different undergraduate institutions. The goal of these programs is to give highly qualified high school students an opportunity to broaden their premedical preparation without having to compete for admission to medical school.

About the BA-MD Program:

Students accepted into this program must maintain an overall minimum GPA of 3.4, and a minimum science GPA of 3.4. Also, students must engage in research at the New Jersey Medical School over a summer during their undergraduate studies. Finally, although no minimum score is required on the test, students must also sit for the MCAT.

Program Title	Joint Bachelor / Medical Degree Program
Length of Program	7-years (three undergraduate years).
Number of Students	No quota.
High School Requirements	SAT score of 1400, minimum required. High School rank in the top 10%, minimum required.
Application Deadline	January 7.
MCAT Requirements	Yes. Not a factor for promotion to medical school.

Undergraduate Institution: **Rutgers University**
Medical School: UMDNJ—Robert   Wood   Johnson
                              Medical School

Undergraduate Contact Information:	*Medical School Contact Information:*
Bachelor/Medical Degree Program	Office of Admissions
Health Professions Office	UMDNJ – Robert Wood Johnson Medical
Nelson Biological Lab	School
Rutgers University	675 Hoes Lane
604 Allison Road	Piscataway, NJ 08854
Piscataway, NJ 08854	(732) 235-4576
(732) 445-5667	
hpo@biology.rutgers.edu	
1999-2000 tuition: $4,762	*1999-2000 tuition*: $16,052
($9,692 for non-residents)	($25,119 for non-residents)
http://lifesci.rutgers.edu/~hpo/	

About the Medical School:

The Robert Wood Johnson Medical School, formerly known as the Rutgers Medical School, is a public institution and is named after its benefactor, the former head of the Johnson & Johnson Company. The medical school has two main teaching hospitals. The first is the Robert Wood Johnson University Hospital in New Brunswick. The second is Cooper Hospital in Camden. The medical school also has a separate division in Camden based at Cooper Hospital, where some of the medical students receive all of their clinical training. The average class size is 145 students.

About the BS-MD Program:

The Joint Bachelor / Medical Degree Program is designed to permit the early identification and admission of high-quality medical students. It also integrates medical studies with liberal arts study. Applicants must be students at Rutgers University and are selected for this program at the end of their sophomore year. During the last two years of bachelor's degree work, accepted students will take one or two medical school courses each semester, some of which will count toward the undergraduate biology major as well as the medical degree.

Program Title	Joint Bachelor / Medical Degree Program
Length of Program	8-years.
Number of Students	12
High School Requirements	Students must be Sophomores at Rutgers University. Students must have completed 40 credits, (at least 30 at Rutgers). GPA of 3.3, required minimum. 5 Letters of Recommendation from Rutgers faculty. Demonstration of maturity and commitment to a medicine.
Application Deadline	June 1 of Sophomore Year.
MCAT Requirements	None.

Undergraduate Institution: **Stevens Institute of Technology**
Medical School: UMDNJ—New Jersey Medical School

Undergraduate Contact Information:	*Medical School Contact Information:*
Director of Honors Admissions Program Stevens Institute of Technology Hoboken, NJ 07030 (201) 216-5193	Office of Admissions C653 MSB UMDNJ – New Jersey Medical School 185 South Orange Avenue Newark, NJ 07103 (973) 972-4631
1999-2000 tuition: $21,140	*1999-2000 tuition*: $16,052 ($25,119 for non-residents)

About the Medical School:

The New Jersey Medical School of the University of Medicine and Dentistry of New Jersey is a public institution established in Newark, New Jersey in 1977. The average medical school class size is 170 students.

The New Jersey Medical School has established accelerated baccalaureate/MD-degree programs in collaboration with different undergraduate institutions. The goal of these programs is to give highly qualified high school students an opportunity to broaden their premedical preparation without having to compete for admission to medical school.

About the BS-MD Program:

As a participant in the program, students must maintain an overall minimum GPA of 3.4, and maintain a minimum science GPA of 3.4. Also, students must engage in research at the New Jersey Medical School over a summer during their undergraduate studies. Finally, although no minimum score is required on the test, students must also sit for the MCAT.

Program Title	The 7-Year BS/MD Program
Length of Program	7-years (three undergraduate years).
Number of Students	No quota.
High School Requirements	SAT score of 1400, minimum required. High School rank in the top 10%, minimum required.
Application Deadline	January 7.
MCAT Requirements	Yes. Not a factor for promotion to medical school.

Undergraduate Institution: **Binghamton University**
Medical School: SUNY—Upstate Medical University
                               College of Medicine

Undergraduate Contact Information:	*Medical School Contact Information:*
The Early Acceptance Program for UMEDS SUNY – Health Science Center at Syracuse PO Box 1000 Binghamton, NY 13902 (607) 770-8515	Admissions Committee SUNY – Upstate Medical University College of Medicine 155 Elizabeth Blackwell Street Syracuse, NY 13210 (315) 464-4570
1999-2000 tuition: $3,200	*1999-2000 tuition*: $10,840
http://www.binghamton.edu/home/academic/prehealth.html	

About the Medical School:

The Upstate Medical University is a public institution and was founded in 1834, originally as the Geneva Medical College. The college joined Syracuse University in 1872. The college was later transferred to the SUNY system in 1950 and was renamed the Health Science Center at Syracuse. In 1999, the name was changed to its current name, SUNY—Upstate Medical University. The average class size is 150.

About the BS-MD Program:

The Early Acceptance Program for Underrepresented Minority or Economically Disadvantaged Students program was established to train primary care physicians to practice in rural areas of New York state. The program guarantees admission for four years at Binghamton University, and four years at the Upstate Medical University for quali-fied high school seniors residing in designated rural areas of the state. The Early Acceptance Program for Underrepresented Minority or Economically Disadvantaged Students offers the same opportunity for applicants from populations that are underrepresented in the field of medicine.

Program Title	The Early Acceptance Program for Underrepresented Minority or Economically Disadvantaged Students
Length of Program	8-years
Number of Students	3-5
High School Requirements	Must be a New York resident. SAT score of 900, minimum required. High School grade average of 85%, minimum required.
Application Deadline	January 1.
MCAT Requirements	None.

Undergraduate Institution: **Brooklyn College**
Medical School: SUNY—Downstate   Medical   Center
                              College of Medicine

Undergraduate Contact Information:	_Medical School Contact Information:_
Director, BA/MD Program	Director of Admission
2231 Boylan Hall	SUNY – Health Science Center at Brooklyn
Brooklyn College	450 Clarkson Avneue – Box 60M
2900 Bedford Avenue	Brooklyn, NY 11203
Brooklyn, NY 11210	(718) 270-2446
(718) 951-4706	
1999-2000 tuition: $3,200	_1999-2000 tuition_: $10,840 ($21,940 for non-residents)
http://www.brooklyn.cuny.edu/bc/offices/admit	

About the Medical School:

The College of Medicine of the SUNY—Downstate Medical Center is a public institution founded originally as a part of Long Island College Hospital in 1860. In 1950, The College of Medicine joined the SUNY system. The average class size is 180 students.

About the BA-MD Program:

The program aims to produce physicians who are humanists, concerned with the caring as well as curing dimensions of medicine, and to offer an economically affordable baccalaureate and medical school education.

Students must maintain a minimum cumulative GPA of 3.5, and a minimum science GPA of 3.5. Students must also take the MCAT during their junior year and score a minimum of 9 on all three sections to be promoted to the medical school.

Program Title	The BA / MD Program
Length of Program	8-years
Number of Students	15
High School Requirements	Preference is given to New York residents. SAT score of 1300, minimum required. (Enrolled students had average SAT of 1400, and a 95% average) Demonstration of maturity and motivation.
Application Deadline	December 31.
MCAT Requirements	Yes. Must achieve a minimum score of 9 on each subtest.

Undergraduate Institution: **New York University**
Medical School: NYU School of Medicine

Undergraduate Contact Information:	_Medical School Contact Information:_
Admissions Office	Office of Admissions
New York University	New York University School of Medicine
22 Washington Square North	PO Box 1924
New York, NY 10011	New York, NY 10016
(212) 998-4500	(212) 263-5290
1999-2000 tuition: $23,456	_1999-2000 tuition_: $23,285
http://www.nyu.edu/cas/bulletin/preprof.htm#Accel	

About the Medical School:

The New York University School of Medicine is a private institution and was founded in 1841. The average class size is 160 students.

About the BA-MD Program:

The BA/MD program is a joint program between the College of Arts and Science and the School of Medicine. The goal of the program is to train scientifically and humanistic physicians and to encourage students to pursue intellectual areas outside of the sciences. Students are admitted to the College of Arts and Sciences as freshmen and are offered admission, at the same time to the New York University School of Medicine.

While at the College of Arts and Sciences, students in this program must complete all the requirements for the undergraduate degree and are expected to maintain a minimum overall GPA of 3.5 and to earn a minimum grade of B in all required science courses. BA/MD students must also complete an interdisciplinary independent study project. Students are assigned mentors at the School of Medicine at an early stage in the program so that they are integrated early into the medical school and the medical profession.

Program Title	The BA/MD Program
Length of Program	8-years.
Number of Students	3
High School Requirements	SAT, GPA/Rank, and SAT II subject test (three) are required. Demonstration of motivation and intellectual curiosity.
Application Deadline	January 15.
MCAT Requirements	None.

Undergraduate Institution: **Rensselaer Polytechnic Institute**
Medical School: Albany Medical College

Undergraduate Contact Information:	_Medical School Contact Information:_
Dean of Undergraduate Admissions	Office of Admissions, Mail Code 3
Rensselaer Polytechnic Institute	Albany Medical College
110 Eight Street	47 New Scotland Avenue
Troy, NY 12180	Albany, NY 12208
(518) 276-6216	(518) 262-5521
admissions@rpi.edu	
1999-2000 tuition: $22,300	_1999-2000 tuition_: $30,797
http://www.rpi.edu/dept/bio/info/biomed.html	

About the Medical School:

The Albany Medical College is a private institution founded in 1839. The college buildings and those of the Albany Medical Center Hospital are physically joined in one large complex that comprises the Albany Medical Center. The average class size is 130 students.

About the BS-MD Program:

The Accelerated Physician-Scientist Program offers qualified individuals the opportunity to become physicians who are intensively trained in medical research. This approach provides a well-rounded perspective that prepares future practitioners and physician-scientists to perform with confidence and care in a technologically changing environment.

Program Title	The Accelerated Physician-Scientist Program
Length of Program	7-years (three undergraduate years).
Number of Students	20
High School Requirements	SAT, Rank, and SAT II(in writing, math, and a science) required. (Enrolled students had average SAT over 1400). Demonstration of motivation, maturity, and capacity.
Application Deadline	December 1.
MCAT Requirements	None.

Undergraduate Institution: **University of Rochester**
Medical School: University of Rochester School of
                              Medicine and Dentistry

Undergraduate Contact Information:	*Medical School Contact Information:*
Rochester Early Medical Scholars Coordinator University of Rochester Undergraduate Admissions – Box 270251 Rochester, NY 14627 (716) 275-3221	Director of Admission University of Rochester School of Medicine and Dentistry Medical Center Box 601A Rochester, NY 14642 (716) 275-4539
1999-2000 tuition: $22,300	*1999-2000 tuition:* $26,900
http://www.rochester.edu/Bulletin/Admissions/index.html	

About the Medical School:

The School of Medicine and Dentistry is a private institution established by the University of Rochester in 1920. The School of Medicine professes the biopsychosocial model of learning that is a student-centered educational program. The average class size is 100 students.

About the BA/BS-MD Program:

The Rochester Early Medical Scholars Program is an eight-year program designed for exceptionally talented undergraduates. Students enrolled in this program enter the University of Rochester with an assurance of admission to the University's School of Medicine and Dentistry when they complete their undergraduate degree programs, provided that they maintain a high level of academic achievement, fulfill college and departmental requirements, and complete required premedical courses. The program allows the utmost flexibility in degree programs, mentoring relationships with medical school staff, and early exposure to medical school curriculum through a series of lectures and seminars.

In the program, students must maintain a minimum cumulative GPA of 3.3, and a minimum premedical courses GPA of 3.3, by the end of their sophomore year. Students must have a minimum cumulative GPA of 3.5 by the time of their undergraduate graduation.

Program Title	The Rochester Early Medical Scholars Program
Length of Program	8-years.
Number of Students	10-15
High School Requirements	SAT score of 1300, minimum required. (Students enrolled had average SAT over 1400) High School transcript with emphasis on Honors or AP courses. Demonstration of character, maturity, commitment to medicine.
Application Deadline	January 6.
MCAT Requirements	None.

Undergraduate Institution: **Siena College**
Medical School: Albany Medical College

Undergraduate Contact Information:	_Medical School Contact Information:_
Office of Admissions	Office of Admissions, Mail Code 3
Siena College	Albany Medical College
515 Loudon Road	47 New Scotland Avenue
Loudonville, NY 12211	Albany, NY 12208
(518) 783-2423	(518) 262-5521
1999-2000 tuition: $13,600	_1999-2000 tuition_: $30,797
http://www.siena.edu	

About the Medical School:

The Albany Medical College is a private institution founded in 1839. The college buildings and those of the Albany Medical Center Hospital are physically joined in one large complex that comprises the Albany Medical Center. The average class size is 130 students.

About the BS-MD Program:

Each year exceptional high school seniors are jointly accepted by Siena and the Albany Medical College into this Eight-Year Continuum of Medical Education that has a distinct emphasis on service. All applications are carefully reviewed looking for those special qualities that are the hallmarks of the program: scholarship, leadership, excellent communication skills, demonstrated commitment to service, and potential for contribution to the Siena College community. The length of service and level of involvement are examined carefully. We are seeking students who have a genuine commitment to serve and not those performing activities for the sole purpose of gaining admission into medical school.

Students must maintain a minimum cumulative GPA of 3.4 as well as participate in a required summer of human service in a health-related agency, usually in a ghetto or developing nation.

Program Title	Eight-Year Continuum of Medical Education
Length of Program	8-years.
Number of Students	12-14
High School Requirements	SAT score of 1300, minimum required. High School class rank within top 10%, minimum required. Demonstration of distinct emphasis on community service.
Application Deadline	December 15.
MCAT Requirements	None.

Undergraduate Institution: **Sophie Davis School of Biomedical Education**

Medical School: City University of New York Medical School

Undergraduate Contact Information: Office of Education Sophie Davis School of Biomedical Education Y Building, Room 205N 138th Street and Convent Avenue New York, NY 10031 (212) 650-7708	*Medical School Contact Information:* N / A
1997-1998 tuition: $3,400	*1999-2000 tuition:* $ N / A
http://med.cuny.edu/bsmd.html	

About the Medical School:

The medical school portion of this program involves the final two clinical years of medical education. Students will transfer into one of seven New York medical schools to complete their medical education and receive their MD degree: Albany Medical College, New York Medical College, New York University, SUNY—Downstate Medical Center, SUNY—Stony Brook, SUNY—Upstate Medical University, or SUNY Clinical Campus—Binghamton.

This program is in response to the continuing shortage of primary care physicians in our nation. NOTE: All students entering CUNY Medical School must sign a post-graduate service commitment agreement promising to provide primary care medical services in a New York State medically-underserved urban community for a period of two years following their residency training.

About the BS-MD Program:

The Biomedical Education Program is designed as a seven-year integrated curriculum. During the first five years of the program, students fulfill all requirements for the BS degree as well as the pre-clinical portion of a medical school curriculum. After successfully completing the five-year sequence and passing Step I of the U.S. Medical Licensure Examination, students then transfer to one of the above listed seven medical schools for their final two years of clinical training. The BS degree is conferred by City College, while the medical school to which the student transfers awards the MD degree.

Program Title	The BS / MD Program
Length of Program	7-years.
Number of Students	60
High School Requirements	Must be a New York resident. Demonstration of commitment to medicine and the under-served.
Application Deadline	January 15.
MCAT Requirements	None.

Undergraduate Institution: **SUNY—Stony Brook**
Medical School: SUNY—Stony Brook School of Medicine
                              Health Science Center

Undergraduate Contact Information:	*Medical School Contact Information:*
Scholars for Medicine Program	Committee on Admissions
The Honors College	Level 4 Health Sciences Center
SUNY at Stony Brook	SUNY – Stony Brook School of Medicine
3071 North Melville Library	Stony Brook, NY 11794
Stony Brook, NY 11794	(631) 444-2113
1999-2000 tuition: $1,700	*1999-2000 tuition:* $10,840
($4,150 for non-residents)	($21,940 for non-residents)
http://naples.cc.sunysb.edu/CAS/honors.nsf/pages/medicine	

About the Medical School:

The SUNY—Stony Brook School of Medicine is a public institution, established in 1971. It is a part of the Stony Brook Health Science Center, which includes the University Hospital. The average class size is 100 students.

About the BS-MD Program:

The Scholars for Medicine Program is a special track within the Honors College, reserved for a small number of students who intend to pursue a career in medicine. This eight-year program was designed for high achieving students who want a solid liberal arts education before entering medical school. Accepted students have access to a wide array of liberal arts courses offered through the University and its Honors College.

A seat in Stony Brook's School for Medicine is reserved for each Scholar for Medicine who successfully completes the four-year Honors College program, who maintains a minimum 3.4 GPA, completes all the required pre-medical courses successfully, and attains a cumulative

MCAT score comparable to the national average of medical school matriculates.

Program Title	Scholars for Medicine Program
Length of Program	8-years.
Number of Students	5
High School Requirements	SAT score of 1350, minimum required. Demonstration of commitment to medicine.
Application Deadline	January 15.
MCAT Requirements	Yes. Must achieve the national average.

Undergraduate Institution: **Union College**
Medical School: Albany Medical College

Undergraduate Contact Information:	_Medical School Contact Information:_
Associate Dean of Admissions	Office of Admissions, Mail Code 3
Union College	Albany Medical College
Schenectady, NY 12308	47 New Scotland Avenue
(518) 388-6112	Albany, NY 12208
admissions@union.edu	(518) 262-5521
1999-2000 tuition: $23,892	_1999-2000 tuition_: $30,797
http://dudley.union.edu/Admissions/Applying/TypesOfAdmission/Medical.html	

About the Medical School:

The Albany Medical College is a private institution founded in 1839. The college buildings and those of the Albany Medical Center Hospital are physically joined in one large complex that comprises the Albany Medical Center. The average class size is 130 students.

About the BS-MD Program:

The Leadership in Medicine/Health Systems Program is specifically designed for students who want to prepare for the challenge of medical leadership by taking advantage of additional educational opportunities as part of their undergraduate education. Program students will complete an interdepartmental major in humanities or social sciences and a special program in biomedical ethics that will prepare them for extensive training in medical ethics that they will receive at the Albany Medical College. Students also will complete a term of study abroad where they will be exposed to the health care systems of other countries and a master's-level program in health care management at Union's Graduate Management Institute. Additionally, while they are at Union, students will have the option of also earning a Master's in Business Administration (MBA) with five additional courses.

Program Title	
	The Leadership in Medicine/Health Systems Program
Length of Program	8-years.
Number of Students	15-20
High School Requirements	SAT score of 1300, minimum required. SAT II scores of 610, minimum required in three subjects. High School class rank within top 10%. Demonstration of an interest in medicine.
Application Deadline	December 15.
MCAT Requirements	None.

Undergraduate Institution: **University of Akron**
Medical School: Northeastern Ohio Universities College
                              of Medicine

Undergraduate Contact Information:	*Medical School Contact Information:*
(Contact the Medical School on right.)	Director of Admissions Northeastern Ohio Universities College of Medicine 4209 State Route 44, PO Box 95 Rootstown, OH 44272 (330) 325-6270
1999-2000 tuition: $4,152 ($9,113 for non-residents)	*1999-2000 tuition*: $11,919 (23,838 for non-residents)
http://www.neoucom.edu/students/admi/AdminBS_MDSchoolFrameset.htm	

About the Medical School:

Northeastern Ohio University College of Medicine (NEOUCOM) is a public institution dedicated to primary care. The College of Medicine maintains its pre-clinical campus in Rootstown, Ohio. Clinical training occurs over 16 local community hospitals. The average class size is 130 students, 105 of which are from the three BS/MD programs sponsored by NEOUCOM.

About the BS-MD Program:

The program is designed to allow motivated and bright students the opportunity to complete their premedical and medical education in less time without the stress of medical school admissions. NEOUCOM offers this program with three undergraduate universities (Akron, Kent State, and Youngstown State Universities), which are all within a 35 mile radius of the College of Medicine. The program is open to all students, but preference is given to Ohio residents. Each university has its own BS/MD admissions committee, interviews and selection process, but there is only one "common" application.

Students complete one application and indicate the undergraduate university or universities for which they wish to be considered. This application is sent to NEOUCOM; a separate undergraduate admissions application to each university should not be completed.

Students in the program are expected to major in "Integrated Life Sciences." The baccalaureate degree will be granted by University of Akron, while the MD degree will be granted by the NEOUCOM.

Program Title	The BS / MD Program
Length of Program	6-7 years (two-three undergraduate years).
Number of Students	35
High School Requirements	Preference is given to Ohio residents. SAT/ACT and High School Rank/GPA are required. (Enrolled students had average SAT of 1330 and GPA of 3.88). Demonstration of motivation and emotional maturity.
Application Deadline	December 15.
MCAT Requirements	None.

Undergraduate Institution: **Case Western Reserve University**
Medical School: Case Western Reserve University School
                               of Medicine

Undergraduate Contact Information:	*Medical School Contact Information:*
Associate Director of Undergraduate Admissions	Associate Dean for Admissions
Case Western Reserve University	CWRU School of Medicine
10900 Euclid Avenue	10900 Euclid Avenue
Cleveland, OH 44106	Cleveland, OH 44106
(216) 368-4450	(216) 368-3450
1999-2000 tuition: $19,200	*1999-2000 tuition*: $30,600
http://www.cwru.edu/provost/ugadmiss/ppsp.html	

About the Medical School:

The Case Western Reserve University School of Medicine is a private institution situated on the main campus of the University. The average class size is 145 students.

About the BS-MD Program:

The purpose of the Pre-Professional Scholars Program is to provide premedical college students with a greater sense of freedom and choice in the pursuit of their baccalaureate degree. Pre-Professional Scholars complete their undergraduate years with a sense of security that enables them to follow courses of study that reflect their educational interests rather than concentrating on activities that they perceive as enhancing their chances of admission to medical school.

Students in the program must maintain a certain GPA throughout their undergraduate education to be promoted to the School of Medicine.

Program Title	Pre-Professional Scholars Program in Medicine
Length of Program	8-years.
Number of Students	15-20
High School Requirements	SAT/ACT and High School Rank/GPA are required. (Enrolled students had average SAT over 1400 and GPA of 4.31) Demonstration of strong interpersonal skills and leadership.
Application Deadline	December 15.
MCAT Requirements	None.

Undergraduate Institution: **University of Cincinnati**
Medical School: University of Cincinnati College of
                               Medicine

Undergraduate Contact Information:	*Medical School Contact Information:*
Admissions & Program Coordinator, Medicine & Engineering Dual Admissions 647 Baldwin Hall Univ. of Cincinnati, College of Engineering PO Box 210018 Cincinnati, Ohio 45221-0018 (513) 556-5417	University of Cincinnati College of Medicine 231 Bethesda Avenue, Room E-251 Cincinnati, OH 45267 (513) 558-7314
1999-2000 tuition: $4,998 ($12,879 for non-residents)	*1999-2000 tuition*: $12,612 ($22,545 for non-residents)
http://www.med.uc.edu/meded/admissions/highschool.cfm www.eng.uc.edu/meda/meda1.html	

About the Medical School:

The University of Cincinnati College of Medicine is a public institution with an average class size of 160. The College of Medicine has established Dual Admissions Programs with five Ohio undergraduate institutions that allow high school students to gain admission to medical school from the start of their undergraduate education.

About the BS-MD Program:

The College of Engineering and the College of Medicine have developed a special program for exceptional students interested in degrees in both medicine and engineering. This program is designed for the unique student whose interests include the knowledge and skills acquired in an undergraduate engineering education and the scientific and personal expertise obtained in medical school. The total program takes nine years: five years in the College of Engineering, next, a one-year co-op with a medical or pharmaceutical industry, and then four years in the College of Medicine.

Students in the program must maintain a minimum cumulative GPA of 3.4, and a minimum science GPA of 3.4. In addition, students are required to take the MCAT during the spring of their junior year.

Program Title	Medicine + Engineering Dual Admissions Program
Length of Program	9-years. (four baccalaureate years and one co-op year)
Number of Students	
High School Requirements	Preference is given to Ohio residents. SAT score of 1280 or ACT score of 29, minimum required. High School Rank within top 15%. Demonstrated excellence in science and humanities classes.
Application Deadline	December 15.
MCAT Requirements	Yes. Minimum score is 27, with a score of 9 or above in the Biological Sciences, and no less than an 8 on any other section.

Undergraduate Institution: **University of Dayton**
Medical School: University of Cincinnati College of Medicine

Undergraduate Contact Information:	_Medical School Contact Information:_
JAMS Coordinator, Office of Admissions University of Dayton 300 College Park Avenue Dayton, OH 45469-2357 (800) 837-7433 premed@udayton.edu	University of Cincinnati College of Medicine 231 Bethesda Avenue, Room E-251 Cincinnati, OH 45267 (513) 558-7314
1999-2000 tuition: $15,530	_1999-2000 tuition_: $12,612 ($22,545 for non-residents)
http://www.med.uc.edu/meded/admissions/highschool.cfm http://www.udayton.edu/~premed/	

About the Medical School:

The University of Cincinnati College of Medicine is a public institution with an average class size of 160 students. The College of Medicine has established Dual Admissions Programs with five Ohio undergraduate institutions that allow high school students to gain admission to medical school from the start of their undergraduate education.

About the BS-MD Program:

This program was developed to offer high school students a special opportunity to pursue a broad and enriching education at the undergraduate level. Students will take the usual premedical coursework, and will also expand their academic and personal experiences to further prepare them to become the physician of tomorrow. The goals of the program are to develop critical thinking skills, to introduce them to health care environments, provide an orientation to medical school coursework, and to develop the skills necessary to succeed in a demanding medical school environment. Students should enter medical school with greater confidence, and a greater level of comfort and maturity.

Students in the program must maintain a minimum cumulative GPA of 3.4, and a minimum science GPA of 3.4. In addition, students are required to take the MCAT during the spring of their junior year.

Program Title	UD/UC Joint Admissions (JAMS) Program
Length of Program	8-years.
Number of Students	
High School Requirements	Preference is given to Ohio residents. SAT score of 1270 or ACT score of 29, minimum required.
Application Deadline	February 10.
MCAT Requirements	Yes. Minimum score is 27, with a score of 9 or above in the Biological Sciences, and no less than an 8 on any other section.

Undergraduate Institution: **John Carroll University**
Medical School: University of Cincinnati College of Medicine

Undergraduate Contact Information:	_Medical School Contact Information_:
Chairman, Health Professions Advisory Committee John Carroll University University Height, Cleveland, Ohio 44118 (216) 397-4381	University of Cincinnati College of Medicine 231 Bethesda Avenue, Room E-251 Cincinnati, OH 45267 (513) 558-7314
1999-2000 tuition: $16,384	_1999-2000 tuition_: $12,612 ($22,545 for non-residents)
http://www.med.uc.edu/meded/admissions/highschool.cfm	

About the Medical School:

The University of Cincinnati College of Medicine is a public institution with an average class size of 160 students. The College of Medicine has established Dual Admissions Program with five Ohio undergraduate institutions that allow high school students to gain admission to medical school from the start of their undergraduate education.

About the BS-MD Program:

This program was developed to offer high school students a special opportunity to pursue a broad and enriching education at the undergraduate level. Students will take the usual premedical coursework, and will also expand their academic and personal experiences to further prepare them to become the physician of tomorrow. The goals of the program are to develop critical thinking skills, to introduce them to health care environments, provide an orientation to medical school coursework, and to develop the skills necessary to succeed in a demanding medical school environment. Students should enter medical school with greater confidence, and a greater level of comfort and maturity.

Students in the program must maintain a minimum cumulative GPA of 3.4, and a minimum science GPA of 3.4. In addition, students are required to take the MCAT during the spring of their junior year.

Program Title	High School Dual Admissions Program
Length of Program	8-years.
Number of Students	
High School Requirements	Preference is given to Ohio residents. The SAT/ACT and High School Rank/GPA are required.
Application Deadline	December 1.
MCAT Requirements	Yes. Minimum score is 27, with a score of 9 or above in the Biological Sciences, and no less than an 8 on any other section.

Undergraduate Institution: **Kent State University**
Medical School: Northeastern Ohio Universities College
                                             of Medicine

Undergraduate Contact Information:	*Medical School Contact Information:*
(Contact the Medical School on right.)	Director of Admissions Northeastern Ohio Universities College of Medicine 4209 State Route 44, PO Box 95 Rootstown, OH 44272 (330) 325-6270
1999-2000 tuition: $6,016 ($10,920 for non-residents)	*1999-2000 tuition*: $$11,919 (23,838 for non-residents)
http://www.neoucom.edu/students/admi/AdminBS_MDSchoolFrameset.htm	

About the Medical School:

Northeastern Ohio University College of Medicine (NEOUCOM) is a public institution dedicated to primary care. The College of Medicine maintains its pre-clinical campus in Rootstown, Ohio. Clinical training occurs over 16 local community hospitals. The average class size is 130 students, 105 of which are from the three BS/MD programs sponsored by NEOUCOM.

About the BS-MD Program:

The program is designed to allow motivated and bright students the opportunity to complete their premedical and medical education in less time without the stress of medical school admissions. NEOUCOM offers this program with three undergraduate universities (Akron, Kent State, and Youngstown State Universities), which are all within a 35 mile radius of the College of Medicine. The program is open to all students, but preference is given to Ohio residents. Each university has its own BS/MD admissions committee, interviews and selection process, but there is only one "common" application.

Students complete one application and indicate the undergraduate university or universities for which they wish to be considered. This application is sent to NEOUCOM; a separate undergraduate admissions application to each university should not be completed.

Students in the program are expected to major in "Integrated Life Sciences." The baccalaureate degree will be granted by Kent State University, while the MD degree will be granted by the NEOUCOM.

Program Title	The BS / MD Program
Length of Program	6-7 years (two-three undergraduate years).
Number of Students	35
High School Requirements	Preference is given to Ohio residents. SAT/ACT and High School Rank/GPA are required. (Enrolled students had average SAT of 1330 and GPA of 3.88). Demonstration of motivation and emotional maturity.
Application Deadline	December 15.
MCAT Requirements	None.

Undergraduate Institution: **Miami University**
Medical School: University of Cincinnati College of Medicine

Undergraduate Contact Information:	*Medical School Contact Information:*
Office of Admissions	University of Cincinnati College of Medicine
Miami University	231 Bethesda Avenue, Room E-251
146 Campus Avenue	Cincinnati, OH 45267
Oxford, OH 45056	(513) 558-7314
(513) 529-2531	
1999-2000 tuition: $6,112 ($12,766 for non-residents)	*1999-2000 tuition*: $12,612 ($22,545 for non-residents)
http://www.med.uc.edu/meded/admissions/highschool.cfm http://zoology.muohio.edu/Premed/Dual.htm	

About the Medical School:

The University of Cincinnati College of Medicine is a public institution with an average class size of 160. The College of Medicine has established Dual Admissions Programs with five Ohio undergraduate institutions that allow high school students to gain admission to medical school from the start of their undergraduate education.

About the BS-MD Program:

This program was developed to offer high school students a special opportunity to pursue a broad and enriching education at the undergraduate level. Students will take the usual premedical coursework, and will also expand their academic and personal experiences to further prepare them to become the physician of tomorrow. The goals of the program are to develop critical thinking skills, to introduce them to health care environments, provide an orientation to medical school coursework, and to develop the skills necessary to succeed in a demanding medical school environment. Students should enter medical school with greater confidence, and a greater level of comfort and maturity.

Students in the program must maintain a minimum cumulative GPA of 3.4, and a minimum science GPA of 3.4. In addition, students are required to take the MCAT during the spring of their junior year.

Program Title	High School Dual Admissions Program
Length of Program	8-years.
Number of Students	
High School Requirements	Preference is given to Ohio residents. SAT score of 1310 or ACT score of 30, minimum required. High School Rank within top 10%. Demonstrated excellence in science and humanities classes.
Application Deadline	December 1.
MCAT Requirements	Yes. Minimum score is 27, with a score of 9 or above in the Biological Sciences, and no less than an 8 on any other section.

Undergraduate Institution: **Ohio State University**
Medical School: Ohio State University
                              College of Medicine and Public Health

Undergraduate Contact Information:	*Medical School Contact Information:*
Office of Admissions	Admissions Committee
Ohio State University	270-A Meiling Hall
Lincoln Tower, 3rd Floor	OSU College of Medicine
1800 Cannon Drive	370 West Ninth Avenue
Columbus, OH 43210	Columbus, OH 43210
admiss-med@osu.edu	(614) 292-7137
(614) 292-9444	
1999-2000 tuition: $4,383 ($12,732 for non-residents)	*1999-2000 tuition*: $12,771 ($33,786 for non-residents)
http://medicine.osu.edu/admissions/earlyPathways.htm	

About the Medical School:

The Ohio State University College of Medicine and Public Health is a public institution founded in 1914. The average class size is 210 students.

About the BS-MD Program:

The Early Admission Pathway provides early entrance for a select group of National Merit and National Achievement Finalists. This program affords the participant the opportunity to enter the College of Medicine and Public Health after three years of undergraduate study. The BS degree will be awarded after the successful completion of the first year of medical school.

Accepted students will not be required to take the MCAT. In addition, the accepted students will have the option of spending a fourth year to complete their undergraduate studies. Students are required to maintain a minimum cumulative GPA of 3.5. Finally, accepted students will be admitted into the University Honors affiliation program and benefit from all of its privileges.

Program Title	Early Admission Pathway
Length of Program	7-years (three undergraduate years).
Number of Students	
High School Requirements	Must be a National Merit, National Achievement, or National Hispanic Finalist, who has designated Ohio State University as their first-choice institution with the National Merit Corporation. Must be approved for University Honors affiliation.
Application Deadline	March 1.
MCAT Requirements	None.

Undergraduate Institution: **Xavier University**
Medical School: University of Cincinnati College of Medicine

Undergraduate Contact Information:	*Medical School Contact Information*:
Coordinator, Pre-professional Health Advising Biology Department 3800 Victory Parkway Cincinnati, Ohio 45207-4331 (513) 745-3691	University of Cincinnati College of Medicine 231 Bethesda Avenue, Room E-251 Cincinnati, OH 45267 (513) 558-7314
1999-2000 tuition: $15,880	*1999-2000 tuition*: $12,612 ($22,545 for non-residents)
http://www.med.uc.edu/meded/admissions/highschool.cfm	

About the Medical School:

The University of Cincinnati College of Medicine is a public institution with an average class size of 160 students. The College of Medicine has established Dual Admissions Programs with five Ohio undergraduate institutions that allow high school students to gain admission to medical school from the start of their undergraduate education.

About the BS-MD Program:

This program was developed to offer high school students a special opportunity to pursue a broad and enriching education at the undergraduate level. Students will take the usual premedical coursework, and will also expand their academic and personal experiences to further prepare them to become the physician of tomorrow. The goals of the program are to develop critical thinking skills, to introduce them to health care environments, provide an orientation to medical school coursework, and to develop the skills necessary to succeed in a demanding medical school environment. Students should enter medical school with greater confidence, and a greater level of comfort and maturity.

Students in the program must maintain a minimum cumulative GPA of 3.4, and a minimum science GPA of 3.4. In addition, students are required to take the MCAT during the spring of their junior year.

Program Title	High School Dual Admissions Program
Length of Program	8-years.
Number of Students	
High School Requirements	Preference is given to Ohio residents. The SAT/ACT and High School Rank/GPA are required.
Application Deadline	December 1.
MCAT Requirements	Yes. Minimum score is 27, with a score of 9 or above in the Biological Sciences, and no less than an 8 on any other section.

Undergraduate Institution: **Youngstown State University**
Medical School: Northeastern Ohio Universities College
                               of Medicine

Undergraduate Contact Information:	_Medical School Contact Information:_
(contact the Medical School on right)	Director of Admissions Northeastern Ohio Universities College of Medicine 4209 State Route 44, PO Box 95 Rootstown, OH 44272 (330) 325-6270
1999-2000 tuition: $3,762 ($7,923 for non-residents)	_1999-2000 tuition_: $$11,919 (23,838 for non-residents)
http://www.neoucom.edu/students/admi/AdminBS_MDSchoolFrameset.htm	

About the Medical School:

Northeastern Ohio Universities College of Medicine (NEOUCOM) is a public institution dedicated to primary care. The College of Medicine maintains its pre-clinical campus in Rootstown, Ohio. Clinical training occurs over 16 local community hospitals. The average class size is 130 students, 105 of which are from the three BS/MD programs sponsored by NEOUCOM.

About the BS-MD Program:

The program is designed to allow motivated and bright students the opportunity to complete their premedical and medical education in less time without the stress of medical school admissions. NEOUCOM offers this program with three undergraduate universities (Akron, Kent State, and Youngstown State Universities), which are all within a 35 mile radius of the College of Medicine. The program is open to all students, but preference is given to Ohio residents. Each university has its own BS/MD admissions committee, interviews and selection process, but there is only one "common" application. Students complete one application and indicate the undergraduate university or universities for which they wish to be considered. This application is sent to NEOUCOM; a separate undergraduate admissions application to each university should not be completed.

Students in the program are expected to major in "Integrated Life Sciences." The baccalaureate degree will be granted by Youngstown State University, while the MD degree will be granted by the NEOUCOM.

Program Title	The BS / MD Program
Length of Program	6-7 years (two-three undergraduate years).
Number of Students	35
High School Requirements	Preference is given to Ohio residents. SAT/ACT and High School Rank/GPA are required. (Enrolled students had average SAT of 1330 and GPA of 3.88). Demonstration of motivation and emotional maturity.
Application Deadline	December 15.
MCAT Requirements	None.

Undergraduate Institution: **Drexel University**
Medical School: MCP Hahnemann School of Medicine

Undergraduate Contact Information:	*Medical School Contact Information:*
Dean of Enrollment Management	Admissions Office
Room 220	MCP Hahnemann School of Medicine
Drexel University	2900 Queen Lane
Philadelphia, PA 19104	Philadelphia, PA 19129
(800) 237-3935	(215) 991-8202
1999-2000 tuition: $16,150	*1999-2000 tuition*: $27,000

About the Medical School:

MCP Hahnemann School of Medicine is one of four schools that comprises the MCP Hahnemann University, a private free-standing academic institution. The MCP Hahnemann School of Medicine is the product of the union of two old and well-regarded institutions. The Medical College of Pennsylvania (MCP) was founded in 1850 as the first medical school for women. The school became coeducational in 1969. Hahnemann University was founded in 1848 as a private non-denominational institution.

The MCP Hahnemann School of Medicine is managed by Drexel University. Medical students acquire their clinical training in the extensive network of Tenet hospitals and clinics, including the Hahnemann University Hospital, MCP Hospital, and the St. Christopher's Hospital for Children. Medical students spend their first two years in the School of Medicine campus, opened in 1992, situated in the East Falls area of Philadelphia. The average class size is 220 students.

About the BS/MD Program:

This program is designed to give talented high schools students committed to a career in medicine the opportunity to obtain their education with less time and cost.

Students spend two to three years to complete the premedical requirements, before being promoted to MCP Hahnemann School of Medicine. Students must maintain a cumulative GPA of 3.45 and take the MCAT the spring before proceeding to medical school.

Program Title	Fast Track BS/MD Program
Length of Program	6-7 years (two - three undergraduate years).
Number of Students	8
High School Requirements	SAT score of 1360, minimum required. High School rank within top 10%, minimum required. Demonstration of involvement in medicine and the community.
Application Deadline	December 1.
MCAT Requirements	Yes. Must achieve minimum score of 9 on each subtest.

Undergraduate Institution: **Lehigh University**
Medical School: MCP Hahnemann School of Medicine

Undergraduate Contact Information:	*Medical School Contact Information:*
Office of Admissions	Admissions Office
Lehigh University	MCP Hahnemann School of Medicine
27 Memorial Drive West	2900 Queen Lane
Bethlehem, PA 18105	Philadelphia, PA 19129
(610) 758-3100	(215) 991-8202
1999-2000 tuition: $23,150	*1999-2000 tuition*: $27,000
http://www2.lehigh.edu/page.asp?page=uprogs	

About the Medical School:

MCP Hahnemann School of Medicine is one of four schools that comprises the MCP Hahnemann University, a private free-standing academic institution. The MCP Hahnemann School of Medicine is the product of the union of two old and well-regarded institutions. The Medical College of Pennsylvania (MCP) was founded in 1850 as the first medical school for women. The school became coeducational in 1969. Hahnemann University was founded in 1848 as a private non-denominational institution.

The MCP Hahnemann School of Medicine is managed by Drexel University. Medical students acquire their clinical training in the extensive network of Tenet hospitals and clinics, including the Hahnemann University Hospital, MCP Hospital, and the St. Christopher's Hospital for Children. Medical students spend their first two years in the School of Medicine campus, opened in 1992, situated in the East Falls area of Philadelphia. The average class size is 220 students.

About the BA-MD Program:

This program is designed to give talented high schools students committed to a career in medicine the opportunity to obtain a liberal arts and medical education while reducing the time and cost of their total education.

Students have two to three years to complete 91 credit hours, before being promoted to MCP Hahnemann School of Medicine. Students must maintain a cumulative GPA of 3.45 and take the MCAT the spring before proceeding to medical school. A BA degree in Premedical Sciences is awarded after the first year of medical school by Lehigh University. The MD will be awarded by MCP Hahnemann School of Medicine.

Program Title	Combined Degree Fast-Track Program in Medicine
Length of Program	6-7 years (two-three undergraduate years).
Number of Students	10
High School Requirements	SAT score of 1360, minimum required. High School rank within the top 10%, minimum required. Demonstration of strong motivation towards science.
Application Deadline	December 1.
MCAT Requirements	Yes. Must achieve minimum of 9 on each of the three subtests.

Undergraduate Institution: **MCP Hahnemann University**
Medical School: MCP Hahnemann School of Medicine

Undergraduate Contact Information:	_Medical School Contact Information:_
Associate Director of Enrollment Mgmt MCP Hahnemann University 245 N. 15th Street Philadelphia, PA 19102 (215) 762-4671 enroll@mcphu.edu	Admissions Office MCP Hahnemann School of Medicine 2900 Queen Lane Philadelphia, PA 19129 (215) 991-8202
1999-2000 tuition: $10,225	_1999-2000 tuition_: $27,000

About the Medical School:

MCP Hahnemann School of Medicine is one of four schools that comprises the MCP Hahnemann University, a private free-standing academic institution. The MCP Hahnemann School of Medicine is the product of the union of two old and well-regarded institutions. The Medical College of Pennsylvania (MCP) was founded in 1850 as the first medical school for women. The school became coeducational in 1969. Hahnemann University was founded in 1848 as a private non-denominational institution.

The MCP Hahnemann School of Medicine is managed by Drexel University. Medical students acquire their clinical training in the extensive network of Tenet hospitals and clinics, including the Hahnemann University Hospital, MCP Hospital, and the St. Christopher's Hospital for Children. Medical students spend their first two years in the School of Medicine campus, opened in 1992, situated in the East Falls area of Philadelphia. The average class size is 220 students.

About the BS-MD Program:

The MCP Hahnemann University Early Assurance Program is intended for academically select and highly motivated high school students interested in a medical career. It assures students meeting the standards of the program admission to the MCP Hahnemann School of Medicine after their senior year at the MCP Hahnemann University's School of Health Professions.

Students in the program must maintain a cumulative minimum GPA of 3.45, and take the MCAT in the spring of their junior year.

Program Title	Early Assurance Program
Length of Program	8-years
Number of Students	4
High School Requirements	SAT score of 1300, minimum required, with no score under 600. High School rank within top 10%.
Application Deadline	December 1.
MCAT Requirements	Yes. Must achieve a minimum score of 9 on each subtest.

Undergraduate Institution: **Monmouth University**
Medical School: MCP Hahnemann School of Medicine

Undergraduate Contact Information:	*Medical School Contact Information:*
Office of Undergraduate Admissions	Admissions Office
Monmouth University	MCP Hahnemann School of Medicine
400 Cedar Avenue	2900 Queen Lane
Long Branch, NJ 07764	Philadelphia, PA 19129
(908) 571-3456	(215) 991-8202
1999-2000 tuition: $15,686	*1999-2000 tuition*: $27,000
http://www.monmouth.edu/%7Eadmissn/mmcs.htm	

About the Medical School:

MCP Hahnemann School of Medicine is one of four schools that comprises the MCP Hahnemann University, a private free-standing academic institution. The MCP Hahnemann School of Medicine is the product of the union of two old and well-regarded institutions. The Medical College of Pennsylvania (MCP) was founded in 1850 as the first medical school for women. The school became coeducational in 1969. Hahnemann University was founded in 1848 as a private non-denominational institution.

The MCP Hahnemann School of Medicine is managed by Drexel University. Medical students acquire their clinical training in the extensive network of Tenet hospitals and clinics, including the Hahnemann University Hospital, MCP Hospital, and the St. Christopher's Hospital for Children. Medical students spend their first two years in the School of Medicine campus, opened in 1992, situated in the East Falls area of Philadelphia. The average class size is 220 students.

About the BS-MD Program:

The Monmouth Medical Center Scholars Program is directed toward students who have excelled academically and who wish to enter the medical disciplines of family medicine, general internal medicine, or general pediatrics.

Students must maintain a cumulative minimum GPA of 3.3 while at Monmouth, and take the MCAT during their junior year. Students spend a one-semester preceptorship at the Monmouth Medical Center during their senior year at Monmouth University.

Program Title	The Monmouth Medical Center Scholars Program
Length of Program	8-years
Number of Students	4
High School Requirements	Preference is given to New Jersey and Delaware residents. SAT score of 1270, minimum required, with no score below 560. High School rank within top 10%. GPA of 3.5 out of 4.0, minimum required. Demonstration of interest in primary care medicine.
Application Deadline	December 1.
MCAT Requirements	Yes. Must achieve a minimum score of 8 on each subset.

Undergraduate Institution: **Muhlenberg College**
Medical School: MCP Hahnemann School of Medicine

Undergraduate Contact Information:	*Medical School Contact Information:*
Health Professions Advisor	Admissions Office
Office of Admissions	MCP Hahnemann School of Medicine
Muhlenberg College	2900 Queen Lane
2400 Chew Street	Philadelphia, PA 19129
Allentown, PA 18104	(215) 991-8202
(484) 664-3100	
1999-2000 tuition: $20,085	*1999-2000 tuition:* $27,000

About the Medical School:

MCP Hahnemann School of Medicine is one of four schools that comprises the MCP Hahnemann University, a private free-standing academic institution. The MCP Hahnemann School of Medicine is the product of the union of two old and well-regarded institutions. The Medical College of Pennsylvania (MCP) was founded in 1850 as the first medical school for women. The school became coeducational in 1969. Hahnemann University was founded in 1848 as a private non-denominational institution.

The MCP Hahnemann School of Medicine is managed by Drexel University. Medical students acquire their clinical training in the extensive network of Tenet hospitals and clinics, including the Hahnemann University Hospital, MCP Hospital, and the St. Christopher's Hospital for Children. Medical students spend their first two years in the School of Medicine campus, opened in 1992, situated in the East Falls area of Philadelphia. The average class size is 220 students.

About the BS-MD Program:

The Scholars Program is directed toward students who have excelled academically and who wish to enter the medical disciplines of family medicine, general internal medicine, or general pediatrics.

Students must maintain a cumulative minimum GPA of 3.3 while at Muhlenberg, and take the MCAT during their junior year. Students spend a one-semester preceptorship at the Lehigh Valley Hospital Medical Center during their senior year at Muhlenberg College.

Program Title	Muhlenberg-MCP Hahnemann School of Medicine **Combined Medical Scholars Program**
Length of Program	8-years.
Number of Students	6
High School Requirements	SAT score of 1270, minimum required, with no score under 560. High School rank within top 10%.
Application Deadline	January 15.
MCAT Requirements	Yes. Must achieve minimum score of 8 on each subtest.

Undergraduate Institution: **Pennsylvania State University**
Medical School: Jefferson Medical College of Thomas Jefferson University

Undergraduate Contact Information:	_Medical School Contact Information:_
Undergraduate Admissions Office	Associate Dean for Admissions
Pennsylvania State University	Jefferson Medical College
201 Shields Building	1015 Walnut Street, Suit 110
Box 3000	Philadelphia, PA 19107
University Park, PA 16804	(215) 955-6983
(814) 865-5471	
1999-2000 tuition: $3,081 ($6,639 for non-residents)	_1999-2000 tuition_: $28,376
http://www.psu.edu/admissions/academics/pmm.html	

About the Medical School:

The Jefferson Medical College is a private institution founded in 1824. The average class size is 225 students.

About the BS-MD Program:

The Premedical—Medical Program is a 6-year BS/MD program started in 1963. Students begin the program in June, immediately after high school graduation. They spend two full years at Penn State, at the University Park campus, before proceeding to Jefferson Medical College to begin the normal four-year medical school curriculum. Students are expected to maintain a minimum cumulative and science GPA of 3.5. The MCAT must be taken during the spring of the second year. The baccalaureate degree is granted by Penn State University following the completion of the sophomore year at the Jefferson Medical College.

Program Title	
	Premedical – Medical Program
Length of Program	6-years (two undergraduate years).
Number of Students	20
High School Requirements	SAT score of 1450, minimum required. High School rank within the top 10%. Demonstration of motivation, compassion, and integrity.
Application Deadline	November 30.
MCAT Requirements	Yes. Minimum scores not defined.

Undergraduate Institution: **Rosemont College**
Medical School: MCP Hahnemann School of Medicine

Undergraduate Contact Information:	*Medical School Contact Information:*
Health Professions Advisor	Admissions Office
Department of Biology	MCP Hahnemann School of Medicine
Rosemont College	2900 Queen Lane
1400 Montgomery Avenue	Philadelphia, PA 19129
Rosemont, PA 19010	(215) 991-8202
(610) 527-0200	
1999-2000 tuition: $15,270	*1999-2000 tuition*: $27,000

About the Medical School:

MCP Hahnemann School of Medicine is one of four schools that comprises the MCP Hahnemann University, a private free-standing academic institution. The MCP Hahnemann School of Medicine is the product of the union of two old and well-regarded institutions. The Medical College of Pennsylvania (MCP) was founded in 1850 as the first medical school for women. The school became coeducational in 1969. Hahnemann University was founded in 1848 as a private non-denominational institution.

The MCP Hahnemann School of Medicine is managed by Drexel University. Medical students acquire their clinical training in the extensive network of Tenet hospitals and clinics, including the Hahnemann University Hospital, MCP Hospital, and the St. Christopher's Hospital for Children. Medical students spend their first two years in the School of Medicine campus, opened in 1992, situated in the East Falls area of Philadelphia. The average class size is 220 students.

About the BS-MD Program:

The Rosemont College is an all-female undergraduate institution. The Rosemont Early Assurance Program is intended for the academically select and highly motivated female high school student interested in a career in medicine. It assures the student meeting the standards of the program admission to the medical school after their senior year at Rosemont.

Students in the program must maintain a cumulative minimum GPA of 3.45, and take the MCAT in the spring of their junior year.

Program Title	Rosemont-MCP Hahnemann Early Assurance Program
Length of Program	8-years.
Number of Students	4
High School Requirements	SAT score of 1300, minimum required. High School rank within top 10%.
Application Deadline	December 1.
MCAT Requirements	Yes. Must achieve minimum score of 9 on each subtest.

Undergraduate Institution: **Temple University**
Medical School: Temple University School of Medicine

Undergraduate Contact Information:	_Medical School Contact Information:_
Health Professions Advising Center	Office of Admissions
Temple University	Temple University School of Medicine
109 Curtis Hall (005-00)	3400 N. Broad Street
Philadelphia, PA, 19122	Philadelphia, PA 19140
(215) 204-8669	(215) 707-3656
1999-2000 tuition: $6,622	_1999-2000 tuition_: $23,708
($11,740 for non-residents)	($28,900 for non-residents)
http://www.temple.edu/healthadvising/medschol.html	

About the Medical School:

The Temple University School of Medicine is a public institution opened in 1901. The average class size is 200 students.

About the BS-MD Program:

The TempleMed Scholars Program provides an opportunity for outstanding students to gain conditional admission to the Temple University School of Medicine at the same time they are accepted into one of Temple's undergraduate colleges. As TempleMed Scholars, students will spend their undergraduate years in Temple's Honors Program, after which they will enroll in the Temple University School of Medicine, leading to a degree of Doctor of Medicine.

Students in the program must maintain a minimum cumulative GPA of 3.2 and take the MCAT during the spring of their junior year.

Program Title	TempleMed Scholars Program
Length of Program	7-8 years (three - four undergraduate years).
Number of Students	10
High School Requirements	SAT score of 1300, minimum required. Demonstration of motivation to pursue medicine as a career.
Application Deadline	February 1.
MCAT Requirements	Yes. Must achieve a minimum score of 9 on each subtest.

Undergraduate Institution: **Ursinus College**
Medical School: MCP Hahnemann School of Medicine

Undergraduate Contact Information:	*Medical School Contact Information:*
Office of Admissions	Admissions Office
Ursinus College	MCP Hahnemann School of Medicine
PO Box 1000	2900 Queen Lane
Collegeville, PA 19426	Philadelphia, PA 19129
(610) 409-3200	(215) 991-8202
1999-2000 tuition: $20,230	*1999-2000 tuition:* $27,000

About the Medical School:

MCP Hahnemann School of Medicine is one of four schools that comprises the MCP Hahnemann University, a private free-standing academic institution. The MCP Hahnemann School of Medicine is the product of the union of two old and well-regarded institutions. The Medical College of Pennsylvania (MCP) was founded in 1850 as the first medical school for women. The school became coeducational in 1969. Hahnemann University was founded in 1848 as a private non-denominational institution.

The MCP Hahnemann School of Medicine is managed by Drexel University. Medical students acquire their clinical training in the extensive network of Tenet hospitals and clinics, including the Hahnemann University Hospital, MCP Hospital, and the St. Christopher's Hospital for Children. Medical students spend their first two years in the School of Medicine campus, opened in 1992, situated in the East Falls area of Philadelphia. The average class size is 220 students.

About the BS-MD Program:

The Early Assurance Program is intended for academically select and highly motivated high school students interested in a medical career. It assures students meeting the standards of the program admission to medical school after their senior year at Ursinus College.

Students in the program must maintain a cumulative minimum GPA of 3.45, and take the MCAT in the spring of their junior year.

Program Title	Ursinus-MCP Hahnemann Early Assurance Program
Length of Program	8-years
Number of Students	4
High School Requirements	SAT score of 1300, minimum required. High School rank within top 10%.
Application Deadline	December 1.
MCAT Requirements	Yes. Must achieve minimum score of 9 on each subtest.

Undergraduate Institution: **Villanova University**
Medical School: MCP Hahnemann School of Medicine

Undergraduate Contact Information:	_Medical School Contact Information:_
Health Science Advisor	Admissions Office
Department of Biology	MCP Hahnemann School of Medicine
Villanova University	2900 Queen Lane
Villanova, PA 19085-1699	Philadelphia, PA 19129
(610) 519-4833	(215) 991-8202
1999-2000 tuition: $21,760	_1999-2000 tuition_: $27,000
http://www.bio.villanova.edu/html/depart/health/medical.htm	

About the Medical School:

MCP Hahnemann School of Medicine is one of four schools that comprises the MCP Hahnemann University, a private free-standing academic institution. The MCP Hahnemann School of Medicine is the product of the union of two old and well-regarded institutions. The Medical College of Pennsylvania (MCP) was founded in 1850 as the first medical school for women. The school became coeducational in 1969. Hahnemann University was founded in 1848 as a private non-denominational institution.

The MCP Hahnemann School of Medicine is managed by Drexel University. Medical students acquire their clinical training in the extensive network of Tenet hospitals and clinics, including the Hahnemann University Hospital, MCP Hospital, and the St. Christopher's Hospital for Children. Medical students spend their first two years in the School of Medicine campus, opened in 1992, situated in the East Falls area of Philadelphia. The average class size is 220 students.

About the BS-MD Program:

This program is designed to give talented high schools students committed to a career in medicine the opportunity to obtain their education with less time and cost.

Students can spend two or three years at Villanova before being promoted to MCP Hahnemann School of Medicine. Students must maintain a cumulative GPA of 3.45 and take the MCAT the spring before proceeding to medical school.

Program Title	Fast Track BS/MD Program
Length of Program	6-7 years (two-three undergraduate years).
Number of Students	10
High School Requirements	SAT score of 1360, minimum required. GPA of 3.6/4.0, minimum required. High School rank within the top 10%. Demonstration of exposure to the hospital setting.
Application Deadline	November 15.
MCAT Requirements	Yes. Must achieve minimum score of 9 on each subtests.

Undergraduate Institution: **West Chester University**
Medical School: MCP Hahnemann School of Medicine

Undergraduate Contact Information:	*Medical School Contact Information:*
Pre-Medical Office	Admissions Office
West Chester University	MCP Hahnemann School of Medicine
West Chester, PA 19393	2900 Queen Lane
(610) 436-2978	Philadelphia, PA 19129
pmed@wcupa.edu	(215) 991-8202
1999-2000 tuition: $1,809 ($4,523 for non-residents)	*1999-2000 tuition*: $27,000
http://www.wcupa.edu/%5Facademics/sch%5Fcas/med/assure.htm	

About the Medical School:

MCP Hahnemann School of Medicine is one of four schools that comprises the MCP Hahnemann University, a private free-standing academic institution. The MCP Hahnemann School of Medicine is the product of the union of two old and well-regarded institutions. The Medical College of Pennsylvania (MCP) was founded in 1850 as the first medical school for women. The school became coeducational in 1969. Hahnemann University was founded in 1848 as a private non-denominational institution.

The MCP Hahnemann School of Medicine is managed by Drexel University. Medical students acquire their clinical training in the extensive network of Tenet hospitals and clinics, including the Hahnemann University Hospital, MCP Hospital, and the St. Christopher's Hospital for Children. Medical students spend their first two years in the School of Medicine campus, opened in 1992, situated in the East Falls area of Philadelphia. The average class size is 220 students.

About the BS-MD Program:

This cooperative program is intended for the academically select and highly motivated high school student interested in a medical career. It assures the matriculant meeting the standards of the program admission to the MCP Hahnemann School of Medicine after their senior year at West Chester University.

Students in the program must maintain a cumulative minimum GPA of 3.5, and take the MCAT exam in the spring of their junior year.

Program Title	West Chester – MCP Hahnemann Early Assurance Program.
Length of Program	8-years.
Number of Students	4
High School Requirements	SAT score of 1300, minimum required. High School rank within the top 10%, minimum required.
Application Deadline	November 15.
MCAT Requirements	Yes. Must achieve minimum of 9 on each subtest.

Undergraduate Institution: **Widener University**
Medical School: Temple University School of Medicine

Undergraduate Contact Information:	*Medical School Contact Information:*
Pre-Medical Program Advisor College of Arts & Sciences Widener University One University Place Chester, PA 19013 (610) 499-4126	Office of Admissions Temple University School of Medicine 3400 N. Broad Street Philadelphia, PA 19140 (215) 707-3656
1999-2000 tuition: $16,750	*1999-2000 tuition*: $$23,708 ($28,900 for non-residents)
http://www.science.widener.edu/pre/premed.html	

About the Medical School:

The Temple University School of Medicine is a public institution opened in 1901. The average class size is 200 students.

About the BS-MD Program:

The Widener Medical Scholars Program offers early assurance admission to Temple University School of Medicine for highly qualified high school seniors. The program has been designed to attract broadly educated candidates who are interested in entering the practice of primary care medicine. Once selected for the program, students participate in a well-integrated undergraduate-affiliated hospital-medical school experience that involves a variety of experiences at the local Crozer-Chester Medical Center. At the conclusion of your medical education, you will be strongly encouraged to apply for a residency program in general pediatrics, general internal medicine, or family medicine at the Crozer-Chester Medical Center.

Students in the program may choose any major at Widener. Students must maintain a cumulative GPA of 3.3 and take the MCAT in the spring of their junior year. After successful completion of major and program requirements, students are promoted to Temple University School of Medicine.

Program Title	The Widener Medical Scholars Program
Length of Program	8-years.
Number of Students	8
High School Requirements	Must be a Pennsylvania or Delaware resident. SAT score of 1270, minimum required, with no score under 560.
Application Deadline	December 29.
MCAT Requirements	Yes. Minimum scores not defined.

Undergraduate Institution: **Wilkes University**
Medical School: MCP Hahnemann School of Medicine

Undergraduate Contact Information:	*Medical School Contact Information:*
Health Sciences Advisor	Admissions Office
Dept of Biology, Chemistry & Health Sciences	MCP Hahnemann School of Medicine
Wilkes University	2900 Queen Lane
Wilkes-Barre, PA 18766	Philadelphia, PA 19129
(570) 408-4754	(215) 991-8202
1999-2000 tuition: $16,362	*1999-2000 tuition*: $27,000
http://www.wilkes.edu/biochs/	

About the Medical School:

MCP Hahnemann School of Medicine is one of four schools that comprises the MCP Hahnemann University, a private free-standing academic institution. The MCP Hahnemann School of Medicine is the product of the union of two old and well-regarded institutions. The Medical College of Pennsylvania (MCP) was founded in 1850 as the first medical school for women. The school became coeducational in 1969. Hahnemann University was founded in 1848 as a private non-denominational institution.

The MCP Hahnemann School of Medicine is managed by Drexel University. Medical students acquire their clinical training in the extensive network of Tenet hospitals and clinics, including the Hahnemann University Hospital, MCP Hospital, and the St. Christopher's Hospital for Children. Medical students spend their first two years in the School of Medicine campus, opened in 1992, situated in the East Falls area of Philadelphia. The average class size is 220 students.

About the BS-MD Program:

The Premedical Scholars Program with MCP Hahnemann School of Medicine is designed to allow early admission to medical school for those students with an interest in pursuing a career as a primary care physician. The program selects talented high school students from northeastern Pennsylvania and the southern-tier of New York.

Students in the program must maintain a cumulative minimum GPA of 3.3 and take the MCAT during the spring of their junior year. Students also spend one semester at either the Robert Packer Hospital at the Guthrie Clinic, or at the Nesbitt Hospital of the Wyoming Valley Health Care System.

Program Title	Premedical Scholars Program with MCP Hahnemann
Length of Program	8-years.
Number of Students	6
High School Requirements	Must be a Pennsylvania or New York resident. SAT score of 1270, minimum required, with no score below 560. High School rank within top 10%.
Application Deadline	December 1.
MCAT Requirements	Yes. Must achieve a minimum of 8 on each subtest.

Undergraduate Institution: **Wilkes University**
Medical School: Pennsylvania State University College of
                              Medicine

Undergraduate Contact Information:	_Medical School Contact Information:_
Health Sciences Advisor	Office of Student Affairs
Dept of Biology, Chemistry & Health Sciences	Penn State College of Medicine
Stark Learning Center	500 University Drive, H060
Wilkes University	Hershey, PA 17033
Wilkes-Barre, PA 18766	(717) 531-8755
(570) 408-4823	
1999-2000 tuition: $16,362	_1999-2000 tuition_: $17,176
http://www.wilkes.edu/biochs/	

About the Medical School:
   The Penn State College of Medicine is a public institution founded in 1963. The College of Medicine was a joint venture between the Milton S. Hershey Foundation and the Pennsylvania State University. The average class size is 110 students.

About the BS-MD Program:
   The Premedical Scholars Program with the Penn State College of Medicine is designed to allow early admission to medical school for those students from rural and/or medically underserved areas of Pennsylvania who have a sincere interest in pursuing a career as a primary care physician.
   Students in the program must maintain a minimum cumulative GPA and take the MCAT during the spring of their junior year. Students also spend one semester at either the Robert Packer Hospital of the Guthrie Clinic, or at the Nesbitt Hospital of the Wyoming Valley Health Care System, as well as two semesters shadowing a primary care physician.

Program Title	Premedical Scholars Program with Penn State
Length of Program	8-years
Number of Students	2
High School Requirements	Must be a Pennsylvania resident. SAT score of 1250, minimum required. High School rank within top 10%.
Application Deadline	December 1.
MCAT Requirements	Yes. Must achieve above the national average.

Undergraduate Institution: **Wilkes University**
Medical School: SUNY—Upstate Medical University College of Medicine

Undergraduate Contact Information:	*Medical School Contact Information:*
Health Sciences Advisor	Admissions Committee
Dept of Biology, Chemistry & Health Sciences	SUNY – Upstate Medical University
Stark Learning Center	College of Medicine
Wilkes University	155 Elizabeth Blackwell Street
Wilkes-Barre, PA 18766	Syracuse, NY 13210
(570) 408-4754	(315) 464-4570
1999-2000 tuition: $16,362	*1999-2000 tuition*: $10,840
http://www.wilkes.edu/biochs/	

About the Medical School:

The Upstate Medical University is a public institution founded in 1834, originally as the Geneva Medical College. The college joined Syracuse University in 1872. The college was later transferred to the State University of New York (SUNY) system in 1950 and was renamed the Health Science Center at Syracuse. In 1999, the name was changed to its current name, SUNY—Upstate Medical University. The average class size is 150.

About the BS-MD Program:

The Premedical Scholars Program with SUNY—Upstate Medical University College of Medicine in Syracuse is designed to allow early admission to medical school for those students with a sincere interest in pursuing a career as a primary care physician. The program selects talented high school students from the southern-tier of New York.

Students in the program must maintain a cumulative minimum GPA of 3.5. The MCAT is not required. Students also spend one semester at the Robert Packer Hospital at the Guthrie Clinic in Sayre, Pennsylvania.

Program Title	Premedical Scholars Program with SUNY-Syracuse
Length of Program	8-years.
Number of Students	2
High School Requirements	Must be a New York resident. SAT score of 1200, minimum required.
Application Deadline	December 1.
MCAT Requirements	None.

Undergraduate Institution: **Brown University**
Medical School: Brown University School of Medicine

Undergraduate Contact Information:	*Medical School Contact Information:*
College Admissions Office	Office of Admissions
Brown University	Brown University School of Medicine
Box 1876	97 Waterman St, Box G-A212
Providence, RI 02912	Providence, RI 02912
(401) 863-2378	(401) 863-2149
1999-2000 tuition: $24,624	*1999-2000 tuition*: $27,704
http://biomed.brown.edu/medicine_programs/PLME.html	

About the Medical School:

Brown University is a private institution founded in 1764. The Brown University School of Medicine was established in 1975. The School of Medicine only accepts individuals applying for the MD-PhD program into the first-year class unless they are enrolled in specific post-baccalaureate programs, early admissions programs, or are a Brown University student. The majority of the School of Medicine is comprised of students in the Program in Liberal Medical Education. The average class size is 70.

About the BA/BS-MD Program:

Brown's Program in Liberal Medical Education offers a unique opportunity to combine undergraduate and professional studies in medicine in an eight-year continuum. The program combines the open curriculum concept of the undergraduate school and the competency-based curriculum concept of the medical school. It encourages students interested in medicine to also pursue other interests (ie, humanities, social sciences, natural sciences) in depth as they prepare for careers as physicians.

Program Title	The Program in Liberal Medical Education
Length of Program	8-years
Number of Students	60
High School Requirements	SAT, GPA/Rank, SAT II (in three subjects) are required. (Enrolled students had SAT scores above 1400, ranked in top2%) Demonstration of maturity, motivation, character, and sensitivity.
Application Deadline	January 1.
MCAT Requirements	None.

Undergraduate Institution: **Providence College**
Medical School: Brown University School of Medicine

Undergraduate Contact Information:	_Medical School Contact Information:_
Director of Admissions	Office of Admissions
Providence College	Brown University School of Medicine
549 River Avenue	97 Waterman St, Box G-A212
Providence, RI 02918	Providence, RI 02912
(401) 865-1000	(401) 863-2149
1999-2000 tuition: $17,945	_1999-2000 tuition_: $27,704
http://www.providence.edu/premed/index.html	

About the Medical School:

Brown University is a private institution founded in 1764. The Brown University School of Medicine was established in 1975. The School of Medicine only accepts individuals applying for the MD-PhD program into the first-year class unless they are enrolled in specific post-baccalaureate programs, early admissions programs, or are a Brown University student. The majority of the School of Medicine is comprised of students in Brown's Program in Liberal Medical Education. The average class size is 70.

About the BA/BS-MD Program:

Selected undergraduates at Providence College, who are residents of the State of Rhode Island, are invited to participate in a program of "Early Identification" which entitles them to seek early decision admission to the Brown University School of Medicine. In the spring of each year, the premedical advisors at Providence College identify those Rhode Island residents in the freshman or sophomore classes who have achieved high academic standing and have demonstrated a serious interest in medicine.

Students accepted in the program complete their bachelor's degree at Providence College before matriculating at Brown University School of Medicine. They are also invited to take up to four science classes at Brown as visiting students. Students must maintain a minimum cumulative GPA of 3.0 for promotion to the School of Medicine following graduation.

Program Title	Early Identification Program
Length of Program	8-years
Number of Students	2
High School Requirements	Must be a Rhode Island resident. Must be a freshman or sophomore at Providence College. Selection by the Premedical Advisor for achievement of high academic standing and demonstration of serious interest in medicine.
Application Deadline	N/A.
MCAT Requirements	None.

Undergraduate Institution: **Rhode Island College**
Medical School: Brown University School of Medicine

Undergraduate Contact Information:	_Medical School Contact Information:_
Director of Admissions	Office of Admissions
Rhode Island College	Brown University School of Medicine
600 Mount Pleasant Avenue	97 Waterman St, Box G-A212
Providence, RI 02908	Providence, RI 02912
(401) 456-8000	(401) 863-2149
1999-2000 tuition: $1,390	_1999-2000 tuition_: $27,704
http://www.providence.edu/premed/index.html	

About the Medical School:

Brown University is a private institution founded in 1764. The Brown University School of Medicine was established in 1975. The School of Medicine only accepts individuals applying for the MD-PhD program into the first-year class unless they are enrolled in specific post-baccalaureate programs, early admissions programs, or are a Brown University student. The majority of the School of Medicine is comprised of students in Brown's Program in Liberal Medical Education. The average class size is 70.

About the BA/BS-MD Program:

Selected undergraduates at Rhode Island College, who are residents of the State of Rhode Island, are invited to participate in a program of "Early Identification" which entitles them to seek early decision admission to the Brown University Program in Medicine. In the spring of each year, the premedical advisors at Rhode Island College identify those Rhode Island residents in the freshman or sophomore classes who have achieved high academic standing and have demonstrated a serious interest in medicine.

Students accepted in the program complete their bachelor's degree at Rhode Island College. They are also invited to take up to four science classes at Brown as visiting students. Students must maintain a minimum cumulative GPA of 3.0 for promotion to the Brown University School of Medicine following graduation.

Program Title	Early Identification Program
Length of Program	8-years
Number of Students	2
High School Requirements	Must be a Rhode Island resident. Must be a freshman or sophomore at Rhode Island College. Selection by the Premedical Advisor for achievement of high academic standing and demonstration of serious interest in medicine.
Application Deadline	N/A.
MCAT Requirements	None.

Undergraduate Institution: **University of Rhode Island**
Medical School: Brown University School of Medicine

Undergraduate Contact Information:	*Medical School Contact Information:*
Director of Admissions	Office of Admissions
University of Rhode Island	Brown University School of Medicine
Kingston, RI 02881	97 Waterman St, Box G-A212
(401) 874-1000	Providence, RI 02912
	(401) 863-2149
1999-2000 tuition: $4,928	*1999-2000 tuition*: $27,704
http://www.providence.edu/premed/index.html	

About the Medical School:

Brown University is a private institution founded in 1764. The Brown University School of Medicine was established in 1975. The School of Medicine only accepts individuals applying for the MD-PhD program into the first-year class unless they are enrolled in specific post-baccalaureate programs, early admissions programs, or are a Brown University student. The majority of the School of Medicine is comprised of students in Brown's Program in Liberal Medical Education. The average class size is 70.

About the BA/BS-MD Program:

Selected undergraduates at the University of Rhode Island, who are residents of the State of Rhode Island, are invited to participate in a program of "Early Identification" which entitles them to seek early decision admission to the Brown University Program in Medicine. In the spring of each year, the premedical advisors at the University of Rhode Island identify those Rhode Island residents in the freshman or sophomore classes who have achieved high academic standing and have demonstrated a serious interest in medicine.

Students accepted in the program complete their bachelor's degree at the University of Rhode Island. They are also invited to take up to four science classes at Brown as visiting students. Students must maintain a minimum cumulative GPA of 3.0 for promotion to the Brown University School of Medicine following graduation.

Program Title	Early Identification Program
Length of Program	8-years
Number of Students	2
High School Requirements	Must be a Rhode Island resident. Must be a freshman or sophomore at University of Rhode Island. Selection by the Premedical Advisor for achievement of high academic standing and demonstration of serious interest in medicine.
Application Deadline	N/A.
MCAT Requirements	None.

Undergraduate Institution: **East Tennessee State University**
Medical School: East Tennessee State University
                               James H. Quillen College of Medicine

Undergraduate Contact Information:	_Medical School Contact Information:_
Director, Premedical-Medical Program	Assistant Dean for Admissions
Office of medical Professions Advisement	ETSU College of Medicine
East Tennessee State University	PO Box 70580
PO Box 70592	Johnson City, TN 37614
Johnson City, TN 37614	(423) 439-4753
(423) 439-5602	
1999-2000 tuition: $2,532	_1999-2000 tuition_: $10,342
($7,648 for non-residents)	($21,080 for non-residents)
http://www.etsu.edu/cas/premed/pmmd.htm	

About the Medical School:

The East Tennessee State University College of Medicine is a public institution established in 1978. The medical education emphasizes primary care. The average class size is 60 students.

About the BA/BS-MD Program:

The Premedical-Medical Program is an eight-year coordinated curriculum leading to both the BA/BS and MD degrees. The Program is designed to (1) identify and accept promising students into medical education early in their college careers; (2) provide a strong liberal arts foundation emphasizing the humanities; (3) eliminate the repetition of some subject matter often present in the usual four-year premedical program followed by four years of medical school; and (4) allow students the opportunity for personal growth and maximum benefit from their undergraduate experience by reducing the stress and anxiety associated with the standard medical school application process.

Students must be freshmen at the East Tennessee State University to be considered for the program.

Program Title	The Premedical – Medical Program
Length of Program	8-years.
Number of Students	15
High School Requirements	Preference is given to Tennessee residents. Must be a freshman at East Tennessee State University. GPA of 3.3 / 4.0 during freshman year at East Tennessee. SAT or ACT score above the 85th percentile, minimum required. High School rank within the top 20%.
Application Deadline	April 1.
MCAT Requirements	Yes. Minimum scores not defined.

Undergraduate Institution: **Fisk University**
Medical School: Meharry Medical College

Undergraduate Contact Information:	_Medical School Contact Information:_
Director of Admissions	Director of Admissions
Office of Admissions	Meharry Medical College
Fisk University	1005 D.B. Todd Boulevard
1000 17th Avenue North	Nashville, TN 37208
Nashville, TN 37208	(615) 327-6223
(800) 443-3475	
1999-2000 tuition: $8,740	_1999-2000 tuition_: $21,824

About the Medical School:

The Meharry Medical College is a private institution founded in 1876, originally as the Meharry Medical Department of Central Tennessee College. The medical school focuses on providing educational opportunities to promising African Americans and other ethnic minority students. The average class size is 80 students.

About the BS-MD Program:

The Joint Program in Biomedical Sciences is designed to address the need to train talented minorities who are dedicated to finding solutions to biomedical problems through research, and who will be future health care providers. Students must be currently enrolled as freshman at Fisk University to be considered for the program.

Program Title	The Joint Program in Biomedical Sciences
Length of Program	7-years (three undergraduate years).
Number of Students	5
High School Requirements	Must be a freshman at Fisk University. High School rank within the top 20%. SAT or ACT scores required.
Application Deadline	December 15.
MCAT Requirements	Yes. Minimum scores not defined.

Undergraduate Institution: **Rice University**
Medical School: Baylor College of Medicine

Undergraduate Contact Information:	*Medical School Contact Information:*
Office of Admissions – MS-17	Office of Admissions
Rice University	Baylor College of Medicine
6100 Main Street	One Baylor Plaza
Houston, TX 77005	Houston, TX 77030
(713) 527-4036	(713) 798-4842
1999-2000 tuition: $15,350	*1999-2000 tuition*: $6,550 (\$19,650 for non-residents)
http://www.rice.edu/prospect/rice-baylor.html	

About the Medical School:

The Baylor College of Medicine is the academic center of the Texas Medical Center in Houston. The average class size is 170 students.

About the BS-MD Program:

The Medical Scholars Program promotes the education of future physicians who are scientifically competent, compassionate, and socially conscious. The program provides selected students with the opportunity to increase their knowledge and skills without worrying that curricular or extra-curricular choices made in college might affect medical school admission. It is the hope of Rice University and Baylor College of Medicine that these students will apply insight from the extensive study of liberal arts and other disciplines to the study of modern medical science. Thus, accepted students are encouraged to explore the entire range of Rice University undergraduate programs to the extent that their interests allow.

Students in the program must maintain a minimum cumulative GPA of 3.2. They are not required to take the MCAT, but it is recommended.

Program Title	The Medical Scholars Program
Length of Program	8-years.
Number of Students	15
High School Requirements	SAT or ACT scores required. SAT II in three subjects required. GPA / Rank required. (Enrolled students were within top 5%).
Application Deadline	December 1.
MCAT Requirements	None.

Undergraduate Institution: **Texas A&M University**
Medical School: Texas A&M University Health Sciences
                              Center College of Medicine

Undergraduate Contact Information:	*Medical School Contact Information:*
College of Honors Programs	Office of Admissions
Texas A&M University	Texas A&M University College of Medicine
College Station, TX 77843	159 Joe Reynolds Medical Building
(409) 845-1957	College Station, TX 77843
	(409) 845-7743
1999-2000 tuition: $2,639	*1999-2000 tuition*: $6,550
http://medicine.tamu.edu/studentaffairs/MSS.html	

About the Medical School:

The Texas A&M University College of Medicine is a public institution established in 1973 as part of the Texas A&M University Health Science Center. The average class size is 64 students.

About the BS-MD Program:

The Medical Science Scholars Program is designed to offer highly qualified high school students, who are residents of Texas, the opportunity to broaden their educational experiences, and explore interdisciplinary programs and projects.

Students in the program have the option of completing their baccalaureate requirements and premedical requirements in as little as two years, or the full four years.

Program Title	The Medical Science Scholars Program
Length of Program	6-8 years (two - four undergraduate years)
Number of Students	20
High School Requirements	Must be a Texas resident. Must be either a National Merit, National Achievement, or National Hispanic Scholar.
Application Deadline	Second week of January.
MCAT Requirements	None.

Undergraduate Institution: **The College of William & Mary**
Medical School: Eastern Virginia Medical School

Undergraduate Contact Information:	_Medical School Contact Information:_
Office of Academic Advising	Office of Admissions
The College of William & Mary	Eastern Virginia Medical School
P.O. Box 8795	721 Fairfax Avenue
Williamsburg, VA, 23187	Norfolk, VA 23507
(757) 221-2476	(757) 446-5812
1999-2000 tuition: $4,687	_1999-2000 tuition_: $15,000
($16,934 for non-residents)	($27,500 for non-residents)
http://www.wm.edu/admission/new/deptsheets/prem.htm	

About the Medical School:

The Eastern Virginia Medical School is a private institution established in 1973 with the commitment to training primary care physicians. The average class size is 100 students.

The Eastern Virginia Medical School currently has combined programs with multiple universities. The purpose is to enlist outstanding undergraduate students into a track that provides greater freedom and choice in the pursuit of a baccalaureate and medical degree.

About the BS-MD Program:

Students interested in the Early Assurance Program must apply after their first semester of freshman year. Accepted students must maintain a minimum cumulative GPA of 3.2 and complete their baccalaureate requirements for promotion to the Eastern Virginia Medical School. The MCAT is not required.

Program Title	Early Assurance Program
Length of Program	8-years.
Number of Students	10-15
Undergraduate Requirements	Must be a freshman at the College of William and Mary. Demonstration of maturity and commitment to pursue medicine.
Application Deadline	December of Freshman year.
MCAT Requirements	None.

Undergraduate Institution: **Hampden-Sydney College**
Medical School: Eastern Virginia Medical School

Undergraduate Contact Information:	*Medical School Contact Information:*
Health Sciences Advisory Committee Department of Biological Sciences Hampden-Sydney College Hampden-Sydney, VA 23943 (804) 223-6000	Office of Admissions Eastern Virginia Medical School 721 Fairfax Avenue Norfolk, VA 23507 (757) 446-5812
1999-2000 tuition: $16,531	*1999-2000 tuition*: $$15,000 ($27,500 for non-residents)
http://biology.hsc.edu/programs.html	

About the Medical School:

The Eastern Virginia Medical School is a private institution established in 1973 with the commitment to training primary care physicians. The average class size is 100 students.

The Eastern Virginia Medical School currently has combined programs with multiple universities. The purpose is to enlist outstanding undergraduate students into a track that provides greater freedom and choice in the pursuit of a baccalaureate and medical degree.

About the BS/MD Program:

Students are selected based upon the merit of both their academic performance in high school and in their first year of college at Hampden-Sydney College. Students selected for this early acceptance are expected to maintain a rigorous academic program as they finish their bachelor degree and are encouraged to take a broad range of courses in keeping with the traditions of Hampden-Sydney. This program affords these students greater opportunities within the liberal arts experience while eliminating detrimental competitive influences associated with per-medical tracks.

Program Title	Joint BS/MD Program
Length of Program	8-years.
Number of Students	2
High School Requirements	Must be a freshman at Hampden-Sydney College. Demonstration of maturity and commitment to pursue medicine.
Application Deadline	December of freshman year.
MCAT Requirements	None.

Undergraduate Institution: **Old Dominion University**
Medical School: Eastern Virginia Medical School

Undergraduate Contact Information:	_Medical School Contact Information:_
Advisor, E&T/MD Program	Office of Admissions
Dean's Office,	Eastern Virginia Medical School
College of Engineering and Technology	721 Fairfax Avenue
Old Dominion University	Norfolk, VA 23507
Norfolk, VA 23529-0236	(757) 446-5812
(757) 683-4078	
1999-2000 tuition: $3,796 ($11,386 for non-residents)	_1999-2000 tuition_: $15,000 ($27,500 for non-residents)
http://www.eng.odu.edu/webroot/orgs/Engr/colengineer.nsf/pages/catalog	

About the Medical School:

The Eastern Virginia Medical School is a private institution established in 1973 with the commitment to training primary care physicians. The average class size is 100 students.

The Eastern Virginia Medical School currently has combined programs with multiple universities. The purpose is to enlist outstanding undergraduate students into a track that provides greater freedom and choice in the pursuit of a baccalaureate and medical degree.

About the BS/MD Program:

This program provides a select group of students the opportunity to pursue an engineering education supplemented by unique medical research experiences in order to prepare them for medical school. From those who successfully complete their freshman and sophomore years, a selected group will be given guaranteed positions at the Eastern Virginia Medical School. Contingent upon completion of the BS program at Old Dominion University, students will automatically enter

Eastern Virginia Medical School, thus reducing the academic pressure of preparing for entrance into medical school.

Students in the program must complete a BS in engineering or engineering technology. A minimum cumulative GPA of 3.5 must be maintained for promotion to the medical school.

Program Title	
	Engineering & Technology / Medical Doctor Program
Length of Program	8-years.
Number of Students	
High School Requirements	SAT score of 1250, minimum required. GPA of 3.5 / 4.0, minimum required. High School rank within top 10%.
Application Deadline	March 1.
MCAT Requirements	None.

Undergraduate Institution: **Virginia Commonwealth University**
Medical School: Virginia   Commonwealth   University
                              School of Medicine

Undergraduate Contact Information:	*Medical School Contact Information:*
Director, University Honors Program	Office of Admissions
Virginia Commonwealth University	VCU School of Medicine
PO Box 843010	PO Box 980565
Richmond, VA 23284	Richmond, VA 23298
(804) 828-1803	(804) 828-9629
1999-2000 tuition: $2,492	*1999-2000 tuition:* $10,428
($11,946 for non-residents)	($26,734 for non-residents)
http://www.vcu.edu/honors/guaranteed.html	

About the Medical School:

The Virginia Commonwealth University School of Medicine is a public institution, originally founded in 1838 as the Medical College of Virginia. The School of Medicine is situated in downtown Richmond in the Medical College of Virginia campus, which also houses the other schools of health professions. The average class size is 170 students.

About the BS-MD Program:

The Guaranteed Admission Program offers academically capable, highly focused students an opportunity to pursue intellectually challenging programs of study without the pressure of competing further for medical school admission. Close contact with the School of Medicine throughout the undergraduate program aids students in testing their career choice and in preparing for a lifelong commitment to learning in the profession.

Accepted students will participate in the Honors Program and are required to maintain a minimum cumulative GPA of 3.5 and fulfill all of their baccalaureate requirements before promotion to the medical school.

Program Title	Guaranteed Admissions Program in Medicine
Length of Program	8-years.
Number of Students	15
High School Requirements	SAT score of 1270 on one sitting, minimum required. Or, ACT score of 29, minimum required. GPA of 3.0 / 4.0, minimum required. (Enrolled students had average SAT of 1420, and GPA of 3.8) Demonstration of health-care related activities.
Application Deadline	December 15.
MCAT Requirements	None.

Undergraduate Institution: **University of Wisconsin**
Medical School: University of Wisconsin Medical School

Undergraduate Contact Information:	_Medical School Contact Information:_
Medical Scholars Program University of Wisconsin Medical School 1300 University Avenue Madison, WI 53706 (608) 263-7561	(Same as on Left)
1999-2000 tuition: $3,737	_1999-2000 tuition_: $16,558
http://www.medsch.wisc.edu/education/msp/msp.html	

About the Medical School:

The University of Wisconsin Medical School is a public institution founded in 1907. The Medical School is located in the University of Wisconsin Center for Health Sciences, which also includes the University Hospital and Clinics, in Madison. The average class size is 140 students.

About the BS-MD Program:

The goal of the Medical Scholars Program is to attract outstanding Wisconsin high school graduates to the University of Wisconsin Medical School. Accepted students are part of the medical school community and participate in specially designed basic science and clinical experiences.

Accepted students have three to five years to complete their baccalaureate requirements. Students must maintain a minimum cumulative GPA of 3.0, and a minimum science/math GPA of 3.6. The MCAT is not required.

Program Title	Medical Scholars Program
Length of Program	8-years.
Number of Students	50
High School Requirements	Must be a Wisconsin resident. SAT score of 1300 or ACT score of 30, minimum required. GPA of 3.8 / 4.0, minimum required. High School Rank within top 5%. (An interview is not required).
Application Deadline	January 15.
MCAT Requirements	None.

ABOUT THE AUTHOR

ASIF M. ILYAS was born in the state of Maryland. At the age of four, his family moved to Pennsylvania where he has lived ever since. Upon graduating from Whitehall High School, Dr Ilyas was accepted into a number of Medical School Early Admission Programs. After much deliberation, he decided to attend the program sponsored by Wilkes University in Wilkes-Barre, and MCP Hahnemann School of Medicine in Philadelphia. Eight years, a BS degree, a wife, and an MD degree later, Dr Ilyas has moved on to the most recent chapter of his life, a surgical residency training program. Currently, he is pursuing training in Orthopaedic Surgery at Temple University Hospital in Philadelphia.

Dr Ilyas's interest in the topic of Medical School Early Admission Programs has stemmed from his own positive experiences as well as in response to the frustration he has seen in many of his friends and family who have been struggling to enter the noble field of medicine. He holds the premise that if this book helps just one committed individual to achieve the huge honor of becoming a physician, his efforts have been worthwhile.